nas

Geriatric Nursi

nas

nas

Geriatric Nursing
A Concise Nursing Text

Alison M.F. Storrs SRN, SCM
Nursing Officer, Highlands House
Royal Tunbridge Wells, England

Third Edition

Baillière Tindall London Philadelphia Toronto
Mexico City Rio de Janeiro Sydney Tokyo Hong Kong

Baillière Tindall   1 St Anne's Road
W.B. Saunders   Eastbourne, East Sussex BN21 3UN, England

West Washington Square
Philadelphia, PA 19105, USA

1Goldthorne Avenue
Toronto, Ontario M8Z 5T9, Canada

Apartado 26370—Cedro 512
Mexico 4, DF Mexico

Rua Evaristo da Veiga, 55, 20° andar
Rio de Janeiro — RJ, Brazil

ABP Australia Ltd, 44–50 Waterloo Road
North Ryde, NSW 2113, Australia

Ichibancho Central Building, 22–1 Ichibancho
Chiyoda-ku, Tokyo 102, Japan

10/fl, Inter-Continental Plaza, 94 Granville Road
Tsim Sha Tsui East, Kowloon, Hong Kong

First published 1976
Second edition 1980
   Reprinted 1981, 1982
Third edition 1985

Typeset by Inforum Ltd, Portsmouth
Printed and bound in Great Britain by
William Clowes Ltd, Beccles and London

British Library Cataloguing in Publication Data

Storrs, Alison M.F.
   Geriatric nursing.—3rd ed.—(Nurses'
   aids series)
   1. Geriatric nursing
   I. Title   II. Series
   610.73'65   RC954

ISBN 0 7020 1059 6

Contents

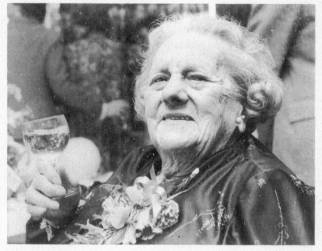

A century of achievement

Preface

This book is written mainly for nurses in training, both students and pupils, for use while undertaking their geriatric module. It is also intended for those studying the English National Board courses on 'Care of the Elderly', and for nurses working within the community. With the increase in the elderly population I hope too that it will continue to be of interest to those working in the fields of general medicine, surgery and orthopaedics who will inevitably meet a large number of elderly patients.

This third edition is written within the broad framework of the nursing process. Emphasis has been placed upon the elderly person as an individual for whom an individual plan of care has to be made. Attention has been paid to the fit elderly and their preparation for retirement, and the care of the elderly in the community. With the sharp rise in the older elderly predicted by the end of the century, attention has been paid to the care of the elderly in continuing care areas and homes, with the emphasis being placed upon the elderly person living as active a life as possible as part of a community, despite some of the disadvantages associated with being old. The role of the carers has been considered, as has the role of the nurse in supporting these people.

Although a brief outline of the common diseases of old age has been included, more importance has been placed on the nursing care of these patients and the role of the nurse in the rehabilitation team. The nurse must be aware of the role of other therapists so that their work can continue 24 hours a day. Although the skills and attitudes required are learned on the wards and not from books, the text includes, wherever possible, practical guidance and detail on assisting the patient to overcome the difficulties which hinder rehabilitation and to achieve the maximum mobility and independence. The chapters on the maintenance of continence and prevention of pressure sores, two demanding aspects of care of the elderly, are examples of this approach. A problem-solving approach has been adopted but the patient's assets must not be overlooked. Caring for the elderly is a

demanding and exciting field of nursing, with room for innovation and experiment for those who are willing to accept the
challenge of improving the care of sick elderly in our society.

Throughout the text the patient has been referred to as 'he'
and the nurse as 'she', purely for the sake of clarity.

I am grateful for the constructive comments and suggestions
made by readers of the second edition, many of which have been
incorporated in this new edition. I should like to thank the staff
of Highlands House for their encouragement and enthusiasm;
Val Longhurst for typing the many additions to the manuscript;
Paddy Mees, Remedial Therapist, for his help and encourage-
ment with many aspects of the book; Dr C.W.J. Ussher, lately
Consultant Physician in Geriatric Medicine to the Tunbridge
Wells Health District; Peter Raymond, Solicitor, for his legal
advice; Alan Doherty of the Nightingale School Library and Pat
Maxwell of the Education Centre Library, Pembury Hospital for
their help in finding many articles and books; Trevor Hill of the
Department of Medical Illustration, Queen Victoria Hospital,
East Grinstead for the cover photograph; and *The Kent & Sussex
Courier* for the photograph facing the first page of this Preface. I
also owe acknowledgement to Dr Trevor Howell for Fig. 3 and to
Professor Bernard Isaacs for Fig. 13. Finally, my thanks go to my
publishers, Baillière Tindall, and specifically to the nursing
editor, Rosemary Long, for their assistance throughout the
preparation of the book.

Alison M.F. Storrs   June 1984

1
An Ageing Population

Geriatric nursing involves caring for elderly people who have physical and psychological problems. It is the unique function of the geriatric nurse to look after the elderly requiring nursing care, but the nurse must be aware of the normal process of ageing and appreciate that only 5% of the elderly are receiving care in hospital and other institutions.

There are a number of words used in this discipline which should be clarified. The word 'geriatric' is derived from the Greek words *'geras'* meaning 'old age' and *'iatros'* meaning 'a doctor'. Unfortunately the word is used freely and incorrectly in such expressions as 'a geriatric chair' instead of 'a chair suitable for an elderly person'. Frequently we hear the word used by the media and laymen in a discourteous and disparaging way when referring to the elderly. However, the word has come to stay and we must learn to live with it.

Geriatric medicine may be defined as that branch of general medicine concerned with the clinical, social, preventive and remedial aspects of illness in the elderly. *Gerontology* is the study of ageing, which is a normal process, but *senile* and *senility* are derogatory words which should only be used in reference to 'dementia' or 'brain failure', which is a special form of mental feebleness rather than derangement, and is common in old age. Senility and galloping senility are not diagnoses and are used rather to hide ignorance than as a true appraisal of the situation. A better word for the ageing process is *senescence*, which begins in our twenties when we cease growing and continues relentlessly for the rest of our life span.

Two other words frequently used in the practice of geriatrics are disablement (or disability) and rehabilitation. *Disablement* is any handicap of a permanent or temporary nature caused by physical, sensory or mental affliction or any defect which prevents a person living a full life as a human being and makes him a burden to himself, his environment or his society. *Rehabilitation* is any systematic activity which helps a person to overcome or diminish disablement and to minimize its social consequences.

Society has stereotypes of the elderly whereby they are denied the feelings and needs that are required by younger people. 'Ageism', like 'sexism' and 'racism', may play a part in our attitudes to people, and although we will nearly all grow old, it is thought of as something that happens to others and we tend to apply different standards to the elderly from those that we apply to ourselves. Old people are frequently viewed as the subject of jokes by the general public and portrayed on television and in the theatre as a subject for ridicule. Discrimination exists in society whereby the elderly are often considered not fit to make decisions, not able to carry out an active job, and very often rejected by their contemporaries for being 'too old'. If old age is not viewed as a time when 'senility' begins, then it is regarded as comfortable and a time for reminiscing, possibly a time for serenity and wisdom, but certainly not glamorous and exciting. Yet many old people have feelings and emotions which they had when they were younger and their needs are similar. Just because we grow old does not mean we are not able to enjoy going out, meeting people, forming new friendships, enjoying a party and doing all the preparation that goes with it. Many elderly do remain active and wish to remain useful to others. They may develop new interests and studies—there are a large proportion of elderly people studying with the Open University and attending adult education classes. Retirement should not be seen as the end to one's useful working life but as the beginning of new opportunities.

Maslow's hierarchy of human needs illustrates that work can help to satisfy the highest need, that of self-actualization. This need is not always met by the elderly. The lowest needs are met by the Welfare State if necessary (Joan Kemp, 1981).

Maslow's hierarchy of needs can be summarized as follows:

Physiological—basic needs necessary for maintaining life, i.e. food, water and oxygen

Safety—home, clothing and protection from danger

Social—the need for loving and belonging, affection and friendship

Esteem—the need for recognition and self-respect

Self-actualization—the need for developing one's full potential; the need to be creative.

Preparation for retirement

Each year about half a million people retire from work (*Growing Older*, 1981). Some do so abruptly, and some retire gradually, preferring to reduce their hours to about 20 per week before stopping altogether. Many are still able to contribute to the world and need to develop their role in retirement. There are some 9½ million people living on state or private pensions in the UK (Eric Midwinter, 1983). Some people now receive a formal preparation for retirement. Many organizations and firms plan their own pre-retirement courses. The Retirement Association of Great Britain and Northern Ireland liaises closely with the Trades Union Congress and the Industrial Society to provide help for those running such courses. Employers and trade unions are responsible for ensuring that people do plan ahead and prepare for a healthy retirement. Courses should cover the following subjects:

- Maintaining health
- Fitness and mobility
- Constructive use of leisure and further education
- Social security benefits and other financial questions
- Housing needs and the problems of house maintenance

Many elderly people join a voluntary organization when they retire and they are then able to use their considerable skills, not only in business affairs, but also in helping those less fortunate than themselves to cope with the difficulties of ageing. Visiting friends and neighbours can help reduce loneliness and isolation.

Some organizations actively encourage the employment of the elderly for some skilled jobs. These include:

Age Concern Link Opportunities — wide range of services from plumbing to entertaining

The Retired Executives Action Clearing House — puts people in touch with voluntary organizations needing help with book-keeping, etc.

The Employment Fellowship — promotes the development of light employment for old people.

A healthy old age

Much depends on the ability of the elderly to continue some form of interest or activity. Many people look back over the past and enjoy their memories. Some can view these with happiness, some are bitter and angry over their achievements or lack of them, and all this has considerable bearing on their outlook on life. Many elderly tend to consider life to have been harder in their youth than it is now and therefore they are not critical of the services they currently receive, i.e. their treatment by social services and the National Health Service, despite the fact that it is often inadequate.

For many people their state of health in old age will depend very much on their life-style when younger; excessive indulgence in food, alcohol, or tobacco may well have a detrimental effect on their health, as will many occupational hazards. Many will retain friendships by joining local clubs and retirement fellowships, thereby keeping contact with former colleagues. Travel and holidays may have been greatly enjoyed by some who feel no longer able to cope financially with these after retirement. However, some tour operators make special concessions for pensioners. British Rail offer a greatly reduced Travelcard and many bus companies also offer great concessions. Recreational facilities at reduced fees are available to many elderly. Libraries cater for those lacking transport by offering mobile facilities in many areas, and they may provide large-print books for those with visual difficulties. Adult education classes are run in many towns and villages, some providing special classes for the elderly who may wish to attend.

Finally, death must come to all, though present society regards this as a subject that should not be discussed, just as the Victorians regarded sex. Yet it is the one thing that is definite in life—we must all die; most of us will grow old and many disadvantaged, and yet few will discuss this openly. Indeed, many of us actively spend many hours trying to disguise the effects of ageing! To come to terms with one's death is of great importance and many of the elderly need help to do this. It is important and necessary for the elderly to recall the past and dwell upon it, and many need us to help them to do this. Many of us too will learn from these experiences. Death should be dignified and not the morbid ritual it so often is at present.

When considering a healthy old age, we must consider the many people well into their seventies, eighties and nineties who are still making an active contribution to life. There are many distinguished elderly members of the Royal Family, politicians and actors, for example, who are still adding dignity and much wisdom to our lives, and from whom society has a lot to learn.

In the Third World the expectation of life at birth is only 54 years compared with about 72 years in Europe, so the problem of caring for the elderly is not so great. Families are large and the children are expected to look after their elderly parents, so they all tend to live together, the elderly parent being regarded with great awe and his opinions sought and followed. This respect for the elderly is very apparent in most Third World countries.

The elderly population

The nurse should be aware of some of the problems of the growing numbers of the elderly and of the care that they should receive both in the community and in hospital when in need. These problems will increase with the increasing rise in the expectation of life at birth over the century (see Fig. 1).

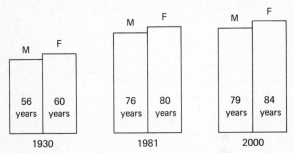

Figure 1. Expectation of life at birth for 1930, 1981 and the year 2000.

The growing number of the elderly in the community is illustrated in Fig. 2, and the expected continuing rise emphasizes the need to plan for the future and for a healthier old age.

The projections for the future illustrated in Fig. 3 clearly show the increased number of old or elderly who will be living longer. The number of elderly living around the year 2000 will be about 10 million, but the number of those over 75 will have risen to 4 million. It is interesting to note that the number of centenarians has risen markedly from 140 in 1951 to 2420 in 1971 to possibly 4000 by 1999 (Eric Midwinter, 1983).

The nurse should first consider the ageing process before

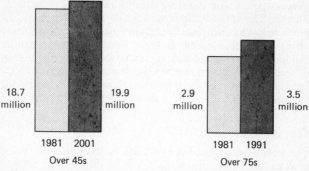

Figure 2. The rising number of elderly in the community.

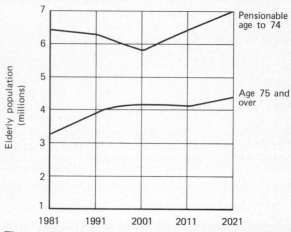

Figure 3. The distribution of the older elderly in the community at the present time and projected into the future (based on figures from OPCS)

considering all the problems and illnesses associated with old age.

THE AGEING PROCESS

The rate of this process varies from individual to individual, from organ to organ and even from cell type to cell type. Individual differences arise not only from heredity, but also from the environment and the ravages of life, both physical and mental. This process occurs in all of us after we reach the peak of growth in our early twenties. From this time on the states of 'active growth' and 'involution' vary as we grow older. The degenerative processes gradually take over and continue at a faster rate than active growth. None the less, active growth does continue to some degree through our life span—injuries heal, blood cells are replaced, and the heart will hypertrophy in hypertension.

Physical changes
The tendency with age is to grow lighter and become smaller in build. The posture is that of flexion, with the head held forward, the spine bowed, and the hips and knees flexed. The loss of height is aggravated by muscular weakness, joint degeneration and osteoporosis. The face becomes shrunken and wrinkled as subcutaneous fat is lost, and the jaw bones atrophy due to the edentulous (toothless) state. Loss of elasticity in the skin makes it difficult to assess clinically the state of hydration. The hair tends to become thinner and may progress to baldness; its texture may become coarse and the colour may become grey or white. Seborrhoeic or 'senile' warts, haemangiomas and other blemishes on the skin are common. Spontaneous rupture of small subcutaneous vessels leads to bruising or 'senile purpura', especially on the hands and arms. The eyes lack lustre and there may be difficulty in focusing. The periphery of the visual field may be restricted, leading to visual inattention. The 'arcus senilis', an opaque ring at the outer edge of the iris, is of no significance. Hearing may be impaired, particularly for high-pitched sounds. Speech may be slower and less distinct. The senses of taste and smell may deteriorate.

Mobility will be reduced and movements such as dressing and undressing will be slower. The gait may become stiff and unsteady, with short shuffling steps. Motor inattention will increase the liability to fall, which is also aggravated by failure of co-ordination and slowed reactions. There may be a coarse trembling or shaking of the head, lower jaw or hands, which is obvious to the onlooker. Poor foot care, giving rise to bunions, corns or deformed toe-nails, may also decrease mobility.

Psychological changes

Almost more important than the physical slowing up is the effect of ageing on the mental faculties. There is usually some decline in intelligence, though this is variable and not noticeable in the majority of old people. Thought processes slow down and elderly people must be allowed to take their time; however, they are able to compensate by drawing on previous experience. Learning continues, although it is more difficult and has to be tackled at a slower pace; practical knowledge is more easily acquired than theoretical. The nurse will often experience this when trying to rehabilitate an elderly patient.

Memory for recent events is one of the earliest mental faculties to become impaired; usually one starts by forgetting names, places and dates. Conversely, events long past may be recalled with great vividness and may be detailed over and over again to the same listener. As a result of this inability to adapt to new thoughts and routines, elderly people like to retain familiar objects and will resist change. They are easily disturbed to the point of confusion by changes in environment, routine and close contacts.

Blunting of the emotions may also occur, with the old person showing no pleasure over joyous events and no apparent sorrow over sad events or bereavements. He may lose all interest in what goes on around him and develop instead an obsessive interest in his own bodily functions, especially bowel habits.

Personal characteristics may be retained in an exaggerated form, and the old person may become a caricature of himself, and fail to conceal his true feeling as he did when younger.

There is therefore a relative preservation of one's intelligence and acquired personal skills into old age. Physical and mental deterioration are balanced by gains in wisdom and experience; serenity should follow withdrawal from the stresses and strains of everyday life. The elderly need peace and quiet, often preferring to be left alone, to give them the opportunity of adjusting to the process of growing old and reorganizing their lives to suit a different pace of living.

Social problems

As many elderly people are among the most deprived members of the community, both financially and socially, the discipline of geriatric medicine must frequently involve social medicine. In the United Kingdom the married couple's pension is very much less than half the industrial wage and 2 million pensioners rely on supplementary benefit, while ¾ million are entitled to draw it but fail to do so. Old people also tend to live in below-average housing conditions. It is estimated that by the end of the 1980s 3 million will live alone, while 23% of the over 80s have no inside lavatory and 20% no bath or shower. Half the houses in the UK without a bath or hot water are lived in by the elderly.

Conditions for the elderly living in the community vary. The most fortunate are those who have been able to buy their own houses during their working lives. However, approximately 191 000 live in residential homes or sheltered housing and some 35 000 in geriatric units or long-stay annexes. Privately owned and rented accommodation so often becomes too large and expensive to maintain when the family have grown up and left home. The houses are often unmodernized and create further problems should the occupant become infirm or disabled. One can see this situation in almost any street of any town or city—the house in need of repair and decoration, the garden running wild due to neglect, the grimy windows and tattered closed curtains.

Elderly people require comfortable, warm, well-lit and convenient accommodation, without steps and stairs. The house should not be isolated—help should be at hand in an emergency. Specially adapted old people's bungalows or flats, warden-controlled flats or 'granny' flats attached to the houses of younger people are ideal.

Poor housing often leads to loss of independence in the elderly, and at present alternatives are restricted. Breakdown of the extended family unit is common nowadays, and in any case the family is smaller than in the Victorian era, when large families helped to ensure that someone would be available to care for the older members, as they still do in developing countries. In addition, the younger portion of the family tends to move away seeking better employment opportunities, and may even emigrate. Employment of women and earlier marriages have also changed the pattern of the family unit. Domestic help has become an expensive luxury, even for the working woman, and it is difficult to get anyone to 'live in'.

It is not the legal responsibility of the family to care for its elderly, but the moral obligation remains, despite the services provided by the Welfare State.

The more one works with the elderly, the more one marvels at the devotion and duty shown by some families to their older members, although households where two, or even three, generations live together, with all their tensions, are becoming less common. Total rejection is rare, although partial rejection may become apparent in a crisis.

The social problems of the aged sick are summarized in Table 1.

Just over £10 000 000 000, or one third of the total public expenditure on the main social programme, is attributable to the care of the elderly.

Table 1.   The social problems of the aged sick

Family strain	27%
Relatives cannot cope any longer	
Nearest relative is ill	
Relatives cannot stay away from work	
Patient unwanted by family	
Disability disturbing home life	21%
Incontinence or dirty habits	
Completely bedridden	
Frequent falls	
Loneliness	15%
Always alone	
Relatives out at work all day	
Mental changes	14%
Confusion	
Nocturnal restlessness	
Wanders and gets lost	
Temperamental or eccentric	
Financial problems	11%
Cannot pay fees of nursing home	
Reluctant landlady	
Financial problems	2%
No social problems	10%

After Howell (1970).

Nursing the elderly patient

Nursing the elderly requires special knowledge and skills and the development of new attitudes and understanding. The elderly patient makes great demands on the nurse, but she will find that the work is immensely rewarding. No aspect of patient care makes greater demands on the nurse's human qualities, her technical skills and energies. Geriatric nursing is becoming increasingly popular because of the incomparable opportunities which it offers for real nursing. The nurse spends more time with the patient than does any other member of the multidisciplinary team, and therefore she is in a unique position to initiate and ensure continuity in the rehabilitation of the patient and a successful degree of independence.

The nurse must remember that elderly people are no less individuals than anyone else and the opportunity to develop a plan of care designed specifically for that patient presents itself when nursing these patients. The nurse must take into account the home life, family, friends and pets, and also the patient's own wishes and fears. Realistic nursing goals should be set bearing in mind the opinions and abilities of the patient.

Nursing within the geriatric unit is a specialty in its own right. Care of the elderly as a specialty in the United Kingdom began with the work of Dr Marjorie Warren in 1935 at the West Middlesex Hospital, and has been carried on by many distinguished doctors and nurses, including Professor Doreen Norton, who since her retirement from the National Health Service in 1982 has had the distinction to be appointed to the world's first chair in Gerontological Nursing in Cleveland, Ohio. Not only is care of the elderly included in every learner's training but there are also two post-registration courses now run by the English National Board—the first run over a period of 22 days intermittently and the second for 6 months consecutively. In 1976 the Society of Geriatric Nursing was set up within the Royal College of Nursing of the United Kingdom and is now a thriving forum for education and debate.

Geriatric medicine too has become a subject in the undergraduate medical curriculum and the Royal College of Physicians now accepts a programme for the training of consultant physicians in geriatric medicine. The discipline of geriatrics has received academic sanction which has culminated in the creation of many professional chairs in the British Isles.

The elderly patient requires a great deal of understanding, kindness and patience, and no aspect of nursing care makes greater demands on the nurse's qualities of humanity, adaptability, temperament and sheer physical strength. Emphasis must be placed less on cure than on improvement to a level where the patient can become independent again and be accepted back into society. The geriatric unit is therefore not concerned solely with the patient's immediate medical, mental and social problems, but with his functional levels, his reactions to illness and the reaction of the family to him, as well as with economic and social problems. The 'total care approach' demands continuity at all levels of care at home, in hospital and after discharge from hospital.

There are many aspects to the problems of the elderly which the nurse should always bear in mind, for she can do much to maintain the patient's self-respect and dignity.

In old age there is frequently a loss of personal pride, particularly regarding cleanliness, and appearance. There is reluctance to change and wash clothing and attend to personal hygiene, probably owing to the effort involved and the lack of any incentive. Feeding habits may deteriorate, becoming messy and neglectful. The nurse must do all she can to counteract these tendencies, although this will not be easy. Many old people become quite out of touch with reality, particularly as it concerns their own disabilities and shortcomings. As a result they will totally reject any help or advice. This trait becomes particularly evident when it is obvious to all but the patient that he cannot continue to live alone and independently. Irritability will take the form of finding fault with everything and everyone. Old people with communication problems often find it difficult to understand what is happening around them; the resulting insecurity will make them possessive of people or property.

The elderly person must be treated as an individual, with a personality of his own, otherwise he will lose his identity and all incentive to go on living. He should be treated like a human being, and not as a mere object which is old, useless and unwanted. To have a feeling of belonging is one of the basic needs, in addition to that for love and affection, which we all share.

The fears of old age are of loneliness and unwantedness and of becoming a burden to one's family. It is important to minimize infirmity when dealing with the old, and this is best achieved by encouraging them to do as much as they can for themselves, no matter how difficult or time-consuming. All these points will go a long way towards maintaining the elderly person's pride, independence and self-respect. It is advantageous not to have too strict a discipline on the wards, with rigid rules. The patients should have some say in their own activities and should be encouraged to express themselves.

The special senses deteriorate with age and problems of failing sight and hearing can create difficulties for the nurse as well as the patient. Inability to communicate seldom brings much sympathy, and this can be most frustrating for the old person if he feels cut off from society. Failing sight and hearing will make the old person withdrawn and further disinclined to accept help, unless the nurse can make the effort to overcome the initial difficulties. It is important to speak slowly and distinctly without shouting, preferably facing the person to whom one is speaking. Toleration of shortcomings in communication is most important.

If they are not kept occupied and out of bed during the day, elderly people tend to drop off to sleep, and are then less likely to get a good night's rest.

Only when working with the elderly will the nurse develop an understanding of their all-too-many problems and difficulties. She must adopt a positive attitude of mind which will help her in the management of her patients and reward her labours. She should not forget the basic elements of nursing care. When working in a geriatric unit there is always the danger of developing a biased view of the elderly, but the nurse must remember that she sees only about 5% of the old people in the unit's catchment area, and these are the ones in trouble with ill health or social problems. The other 95% remain in the community and live their lives happily with varying degrees of help from the community of which they form a part.

Psychogeriatric care

Mental illness is associated with loneliness, deprivation, prolonged physical illness and lack of interest or occupation, and so is especially common among the aged. Elderly people suffer from the same types of mental illness as the rest of the population, and can be treated in similar ways, frequently with good results. The nurse should remember that some 30% of geriatric admissions are suffering from confusion which will subside when physical symptoms have been adequately treated.

Of the mentally ill in psychiatric hospitals 60% are over 65. This is mainly due to the increasing proportion of the population who are over 65. About 1 in 10 old people are thought to suffer from some degree of brain deterioration, leading to various forms of dementia which are so far incurable. Fortunately the condition is often so mild that the sufferer can continue to live at home or in special accommodation for the elderly mentally infirm; for more severe cases the only answer is a mental hospital or long-term geriatric care.

Although the elderly make up only about 17% of the population at present, they account for 33% of suicides, with a higher proportion of men than of women. This may reflect the fact that the social structure of the western world makes it more difficult for an elderly man to care for himself without help.

Paranoid illnesses and depression are particularly common among those living alone. Single old people without relations are twice as likely to be admitted to hospital or to require residential care as are those with families. Frequently the psychiatric disorder may be the continuation or exaggeration of a personality problem established in earlier life.

Hazards of drug therapy in the elderly

There is always a temptation to treat any disease immediately with drugs, but it is easy to make matters worse rather than better by inappropriate or excessive prescribing. In the elderly, drug activity may be modified by a number of factors, including fluctuations in absorption, distribution, excretion and metabolism of drugs. Difficulties in diagnosis, the commonness of multiple pathology and reduced tolerance to drugs due to age or disease all increase the dangers.

Overdosage is particularly likely to occur if the drug being used remains active in the body until it is excreted by the kidneys, because renal function diminishes with old age, even in the absence of detectable disease. There may be a reduction of 30% in the glomerular filtration rate in apparently healthy people over 65.

Complicated drug schedules should be avoided and the minimum number of drugs should be used with the minimum dosages capable of producing the desired effects. The elderly patient with multiple physical illnesses, and possibly mental depression and social problems in addition, is a likely victim for 'polypharmacy' with all its dangers. Moreover, the suicide rate is rising among the elderly, and these are just the people for whom large quantities of drugs may be prescribed.

The nurse can help by asking a patient's relatives to bring in *all* his medications when he is admitted to hospital. Dusty old bottles of all shapes, sizes and contents, and in various states of depletion, will accumulate in drawers, on mantelpieces and on bedside tables in any home. It must be remembered that drugs are the patient's own property and wherever possible permission should be sought to dispose of them. Leftovers should be destroyed to prevent self-medication at a later date or the handing on of medicines to friends and neighbours. A look round the home does not take long and is a useful exercise in preventive medicine, whether it is done by the relatives of the patient, the nurse or the doctor. In addition this will make it easy to ensure that the patient is discharged home with only those drugs he really needs.

It is a help to old people to have their medicine bottles clearly labelled with simple and unambiguous instructions. Chemists' labels are often confusing to those with poor eyesight. The nurse should explain the dosages and their timing to the patient and make certain that he understands; she should also write down the details.

Preventive geriatrics

Prevention of illness is always better than cure, and assistance in its prevention is provided by medical and social agencies, of which the nurse should be aware. Many varieties of service are available, such as voluntary visiting of old people, old people's clubs, day centres, day hospitals, geriatric advice clinics and special housing arrangements. One thing is certain—when an elderly person is in trouble, the sooner help arrives, the better are the chances of successful treatment.

There should be more education and publicity about the problems of old age and the services available to the elderly, particularly by organizations like Age Concern. Pre-retirement courses and semi-retirement schemes will help the old person adapt smoothly to a new style of life, at the same time remaining

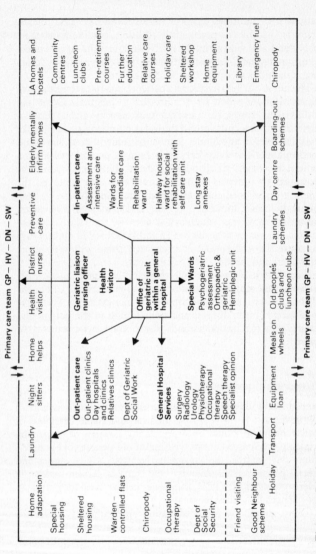

Figure 4. District geriatric services.

mentally and physically active and keeping his dignity and self-respect.

Gerontological research into the natural processes of ageing, and more sophisticated prophylaxis against degenerative processes such as obesity, atherosclerosis and arthritis, will do much to lighten the burdens of old age. The general practitioner and his team of nurses and health visitors should be given more facilities for the screening of vulnerable members of the community, with a view to preventing the occurrence of physical, mental or social crises among the elderly and instituting early treatment where necessary. Health visitors and home nurses are often attached to one or more general practices, although they are employed by the district health authority. Some are based in the general practitioners' premises, while others work from the district health authority clinic. The nurse should ensure that she is familiar with the organization of geriatric services in her area, so that she can give advice where necessary.

If admission to the geriatric unit does become necessary, then it should be as soon as possible; the longer the wait for admission the more difficult will be the assessment of the old person and his treatment and reintegration into the community.

While nursing within the geriatric unit, the nurse must be aware of the role of that unit in relationship to the rest of the hospital and the wider implications within the community. Figure 4 illustrates this well.

References

DHSS (1981) *Growing Older*. London: HMSO.
Kemp, J. (1981) Ageing. *Nursing* (May 1981).
Midwinter, E. (1983) *Ten Million People*. Centre for Policy on Ageing.

Further reading

Agate, J. (1970) *The Practice of Geriatrics*. London: Heinemann Medical.
Copp, L.A. (1981) *Care of the Ageing*. London: Churchill Livingstone.
De Beauvoir, S. (1977) *Old Age*. Harmondsworth, Middx: Penguin.
Tinker, A. (1981) *The Elderly in Modern Society*. U.S.A.

2
Care of the Elderly at Home

When nursing the elderly in hospital, the nurse sometimes gets a distorted view of the sick elderly, feeling that a high proportion are ill, disabled and in need of hospital treatment; in fact, 95% of the elderly population are living in the community, coping well with the problem of ageing. At present the majority of people live in self-contained accommodation, nearly half in their own homes; of the remainder, about two thirds are public sector tenants and a third private tenants (*Growing Older*, 1981). For those living in their own homes and who remain active and independent, it is important that the house is easy to manage, near family and friends, with easy access to shops and public transport. It is important that as the elderly become more frail and less active the home is warm, well lit and easy to manage. Fewer homes now have outside lavatories and no bathrooms, but there are some still to be found in towns and villages, and they are nearly always occupied by the elderly.

The following assistance is available for elderly home occupiers:

1 Rent and rate rebates for elderly owner-occupiers and tenants. The supplementary benefit arrangement can provide cover for all reasonable housing costs.
2 Since November 1980 all pensioners receiving supplementary benefit who are householders and over 70 years of age have been entitled to a heating addition. Higher rates of additions are available to those with severe problems and the basic rate is increased yearly in line with fuel costs.
3 Under the Home Insulation Scheme all householders in uninsulated houses are eligible for grants to insulate their lofts, hot and cold water tanks and pipes. The scheme provides for 66% of the cost to be paid; for those elderly on supplementary benefit or who receive rent or rate rebate, up to 90% of the cost may be met.
4 Grants are available from the local authority towards the cost of adaptation, improvement and repair, and also for improving

the condition of pre-1919 houses, many of which are owned by the elderly. Grants are also available to those who want to improve or convert a house for a close relative.

5 Elderly people can benefit from schemes where the home is used as security for a loan from an insurance company and a life income can be purchased from the company with the sum realized. Since the 1980 Housing Act, elderly people have benefitted from these schemes as well as taxpayers, as they obtain the benefit of a subsidy broadly equivalent to the tax relief which the taxpayer would receive.

6 In some areas now there are 'staying put' or 'Care and Repair' teams operating. These teams operate in various parts of the country and help older people to cope with housing repairs and maintenance.

Particular attention should be paid to the following:

Lighting—	All areas should be well lit, especially those where work is being done. An Anglepoise lamp may be useful for reading and sewing. Stairs too should be adequately lit.
Heating —	Rooms should be kept warm and at a constant temperature. The house should be dry and adequately ventilated. It should be well insulated—some voluntary schemes run by Age Concern and grants may help with this. Hot water can sometimes be heated by an open fire.
Alarm systems —	Many old people now have an alarm system fitted to their house. Some may carry the alarm around with them; some have a bell system fitted in the house. In some cases the alarm sounds outside the house to alert neighbours or those passing by that all is not well.
Furnishings —	For those with a disability, appropriate furnishings are especially important. The right height chair, lavatory seat, and working tops in the kitchen are all important for the maintenance of independence and dignity. Advice can be sought from the occupational therapist. Carpets and rugs should be stable—especially those on the stairs.

Housing associations

In 1977 about half of all housing association tenants were aged 60 years or over. These associations provide sheltered schemes, hostel schemes, and shared ownership schemes where tenants purchase a 60-year lease at 70% of the cost of the property.

Sheltered housing

There is a large supply of sheltered housing now available and this supply is increasing. In 1977 local authorities, voluntary and religious organizations and housing associations in England and Wales provided over 450 000 homes specifically designed for the elderly, over half of them with wardens. Wardens are often resident or peripatetic—they are not there to provide nursing or cleaning. Some sheltered houses have communal kitchens, dining-rooms and laundry services.

Good Neighbour schemes

Many Good Neighbour schemes now exist all over the country, often organized by street in urban areas and by village in rural areas. Help can be obtained on a temporary or even permanent basis for all aspects of home life—cooking, shopping, transport, sitting with an elderly relative, exercising the dog, etc. Such schemes are particularly useful in an emergency.

The aim of good care is to help the elderly in their own homes for as long as possible, and to anticipate the problems and provide support where necessary. When breakdowns do occur it may be necessary to seek the support of the hospital services.

Care at home

Much of the caring carried out in the home is done by relatives and friends. In many cases the help is given for 24 hours a day and can be extremely exhausting and tiring. Recognition has now been given to this fact and many voluntary societies have set up support groups for the relatives, e.g. the Parkinson Disease Society, and there is also a Society of Carers which has set up groups in many parts of the country, where carers can seek support and share experiences. Financial support may be given too in the form of an attendance allowance. Provision for an attendance allowance was made available from 1971 to give financial aid to the disabled living at home under considerable difficulty. Conditions for the payment of the allowance are that one of the following medical requirements be satisfied for a period of at least six months:

1   The person is so severely disabled physically or mentally that he requires another person in connection with his bodily functions, frequent attention during the day and prolonged repeated attention during the night.
2   The person is so severely disabled physically or mentally that he requires continued supervision from another person in order to avoid danger to himself or others.

The following professionals have an important role to play in supporting those living at home and in need of care:

The community nursing service
Ideally the community nursing services should be able to supervise the health care of all the elderly living in a community. The services should aim to keep the elderly in good health, and support the elderly in their own homes using whatever resources are available, whether social, remedial or nursing.

The community nurse
The community nurse is responsible for the day-to-day care of the elderly sick in their own homes. With the assistance of the nursing auxiliary she will assess the needs of the patient and monitor his progress. Bathing, care of pressure areas, drug administration and dressings will all be supervised and acted on where necessary.

The health visitor
The health visitor is more concerned with the preventive side of medicine and may be involved in screening the elderly for potential disease. In some areas an age/sex register is kept and all those over a certain age are visited regularly to ensure that disease is not missed. In some health centres regular checks are made on blood pressure, chest X-ray and routine blood tests. An at-risk register may be kept so that those particularly vulnerable may be visited regularly, e.g. those recently discharged from hospital and those who may be abused.

Geriatric liaison nurse /health visitor
Many geriatric units employ nurses to liaise with the community

services before patients are discharged and also before they are admitted to hospital. This ensures continuity of care so that everyone is aware of the patient's needs and the services required.

Home helps

This service enables people to go into an old person's home and thereby enter into everyday life. It is a support system upon which much depends and the home help can often monitor and prevent a crisis developing. They not only cook, clean and shop, but in some areas undertake more complicated services closely aligned to those given by home nurses. They also provide essential support when the elderly are discharged from hospital and have no close relative to assist them. Charge is made according to income and visits are allocated according to need and availability.

Community care

In some areas a relatively new service, also organized by the social services, has been started called 'community care'. This enables the elderly to be cared for by their neighbours and those living close by, who may visit several times daily and assist with many tasks, and who will be paid according to the tasks involved and time spent.

Provision of meals

This is carried out by the local authority. The meals are either cooked at a residential home or school and delivered by the Women's Royal Voluntary Service, or both cooked and delivered by the latter. The service is provided once to five times weekly depending upon need, demand and availability, and a charge is made. Often these meals are refused by the elderly for a variety of reasons, including poor presentation, repetition of food, inability to eat because of ill-fitting or absence of dentures, or depression.

Other local authority schemes include laundry services, chiropody, holiday schemes, sheltered workshops, boarding-out schemes, advisory clinics, etc. These services vary in quality and quantity throughout the country.

Voluntary organizations

Without the help of voluntary organizations many old people would find living at home even more difficult. These organizations play a large part in caring for the elderly in the community.

Since 1940 voluntary services for old people throughout the country have been co-ordinated and related to statutory services through Age Concern, originally known as the Old People's Welfare Committee, which is represented at regional, county and local level, and is concerned with the care of the elderly in the area. Age Concern aims 'to study the needs of old people and to encourage and promote measures for their well being'. It ensures regular consultation between all bodies and individuals who are able to help to bring adequate welfare service to the elderly, irrespective of their background or income. It aims to provide the more personal services not made available locally by the health or social services, concentrating on providing help, information, advice and encouragement at the right moment. The following services are made available by Age Concern, but not all in every area:

Visiting
Advice and information
Individual services—shopping, reading aloud, gardening, decorating, escorting, hairdressing
Day centres, lunch clubs, social clubs
Laundry
Chiropody
Transport by car, wheelchair or special vehicle
Mobile libraries
Holidays
Outings and entertainments
Housing
Employment and job finding
Exhibitions and competitions
Help in emergencies
Youth help
Residential homes and help with accommodation problems
Aids for the infirm
Day and night sitter-in services
Spiritual aspects
Prevention of accidents
Provision and repair of radio and television sets.

The Council for Social Service also aims to provide services for old people, either directly or through associated groups.

Day centres, social clubs and lunch clubs are all places where the elderly can attend daily, weekly or even bi-weekly in order to enjoy nourishing food and congenial society. Most towns have a day centre where transport is provided, and the elderly arrive in time for morning coffee and leave after tea. They can have a bath and the hairdresser and chiropodist may attend. Entertainment may be laid on, cards, sewing, knitting and conversation enjoyed, and outings organized. Day centres and clubs are sometimes organized for specific disabilities, e.g. for those people suffering from stroke, diabetes, Parkinson's disease or deafness. It is often supportive for them and their relatives to meet others with similar problems.

It is important to help the elderly to continue at work for as long as they are willing and able to do so, although it is difficult with the retirement age tending to decrease. Careful planning should be made before retirement. People should be encouraged to remain amongst their friends rather than to isolate themselves in some beautiful area or seaside resort. It may be necessary to move to a more suitable house or flat with easy access and easily managed heating facilities.

The Employment Fellowship is a small charity whose principal object is to encourage and assist in setting up and establishing sheltered workshops for the elderly. Now there are approximately 100 work centres in the United Kingdom occupying some 4000 old-age pensioners.

Task Force, which is a voluntary youth organization with a local authority grant, operates in London, and similar groups, e.g. Youth Volunteer Action, operate in the provinces, aiming to help the aged and handicapped. Organized by a paid official, they run schemes, often through schools and youth groups, for visiting the elderly, doing their shopping, decorating the house, and gardening. Visits from the young are generally much appreciated by the elderly.

The Women's Royal Voluntary Service provides various services for the elderly. The best known is meals-on-wheels, which is subsidized by the local authority and provides an essential service for many elderly people who are unable to cook their own meals. In many towns meals are available 5 days a week, but in rural areas where transport is difficult the service may be provided only once or twice a week. The Women's Royal

Voluntary Service also have luncheon clubs for the elderly. Some branches of the service regularly visit the elderly in their own homes, and in some cases provide an excellent follow-up service after discharge from hospital.

The local branches of the Red Cross Society also provide some helpful home services including loans of equipment such as commodes, wheelchairs, chairs, beds and walking-aids. They may also help with home nursing for limited periods, providing night sitters and transport if required. They will take the elderly to hospital for out-patient appointments, to visit relatives in hospital and even take the housebound for occasional drives.

Drugs at home

Drugs are a particular problem for the elderly. There is ample evidence of over-prescription, and when new prescriptions are issued, the old supplies are often not removed. Repeat prescriptions are often issued to the elderly without further consultation and as a result the elderly are not assessed and their drug regimen not reviewed (Austin and Parish, 1976). Drugs should be clearly labelled, the instructions must be explained to the elderly person and to the relatives if necessary, and the number reduced to a minimum so that confusion does not occur. Any old drugs accumulated at home should be destroyed where possible to reduce risk of over-dosage or self-administration, always remembering that the drugs are the patient's own property. So often, elderly people living alone forget to take their drugs and it may be necessary to ask the community nurse or health visitor to call and supervise their administration. In many cases, over-prescription or iatrogenic diseases necessitate admission to hospital. It has been estimated that it is responsible for as many as 10% of admissions to geriatric units (Williamson and Chopin, 1980).

Out-patient care

Many elderly can be maintained in their own homes by benefiting from hospital care on an out-patient basis. Some may attend the day hospital and day care and others the out-patient department.

The out-patient department
The increasing load of hospital care is being done more and more

on an out-patient basis. The out-patient department is for those who need hospital treatment and who have been referred by the general practitioner, but whose care does not warrant admission on an in-patient basis. The out-patient department also follows up patients after discharge. This is not usually located in the hospital's general out-patient department, where the unsuitable tempo detracts from the value of the appointment. The interview must be leisurely so that the doctor has a chance to examine the patient fully and is able to listen to any problems that may have arisen. The social worker should be at hand to answer any queries. The majority of patients are brought in by ambulance and therefore may have some time to wait both before and after the appointment. Remember that this may be the patient's first introduction to hospital and first impressions are important.

Day care
Groups in special need:
1 the housebound
2 the lonely
3 the isolated
4 the badly housed
5 those living alone
6 those living with relatives out all day
7 the recently bereaved
8 simple bereaved men
9 the undernourished
10 the handicapped, deaf or blind
11 the mentally frail
12 those recently discharged from hospital.

The day hospital
The geriatric day hospital is a building to which patients may come or be brought in the morning and where they spend several hours in therapeutic activity, returning home the same day. As most of the patients will have to be brought by motor transport, good access is essential.

The day hospital is open daily for 5 days a week and patients may attend as frequently as is necessary, although the majority come on 1 or 2 days only. There is normally accommodation for 20 to 50 patients per day.

The day hospital in a geriatric unit has a marked effect on the morale of the unit, both staff and patients alike, but for it to function efficiently it is essential that there should be complementary day establishments within the geriatric service. These include day centres, day clubs, workshops for the elderly and local authority day care.

The Department of Health and Social Security has estimated that two day hospital places are necessary for every 1000 of the population over 65. It has been shown that, with proper day care facilities, full-time admission to hospital could be avoided in about 1 out of 12 patients. One in 20 would have admission delayed and an earlier discharge from hospital would be possible in about 1 in 10 cases.

The majority of geriatric units have the advantage of a day hospital within the unit, and many of those who do not, have plans to erect one in the next few years. Some are found within the geriatric hospital, some in the general hospital and some are entirely separate. It is usually the central point of the hospital's medical and social services and the heart of the geriatric unit. Some are run by an occupational therapist, some by a state-registered nurse, and some jointly, but in nearly all cases a qualified nurse and therapist are in attendance.

Geriatric day hospitals began in the 1950s when out-patients attended wards or out-patient departments for the day only. It is interesting to note that several psychiatric day hospitals developed in the previous decade. The first purpose-built geriatric day hospital in this country was at Oxford in 1958, but numbers have grown rapidly since then and there are now about 300 day hospitals in the British Isles.

Functions and benefits of the day hospital   The day hospital is a *therapeutic* unit. Its functions are:
  1 functional assessment
  2 medical investigation
  3 maintenance to prevent deterioration
  4 short-term rehabilitation
  5 long-term rehabilitation
  6 support for relatives.

Its particular benefits, in relation to other forms of care and treatment, are:
  1 Treatment for former in-patients can continue in a new environment which raises interest and morale.
  2 A midway stage between hospital and home helps the

patient adjust psychologically to discharge.

3 In-patients and out-patients can mix, which provides social contact.

4 Hospital beds are saved and nurses are released as staffing is required 5 days a week only.

5 The burden on relatives is relieved without removing responsibility.

By far the most important services provided by these units are those of physical rehabilitation and medical supervision. Next in order of priority is maintenance therapy for those who are particularly frail. The third requirement concerns patients needing social care who are too frail to be looked after elsewhere.

Other services available in most day hospitals are dentistry, chiropody and audiometric services (hearing-aids). Ophthalmic opinion in the general hospital will also be accessible on an out-patient basis.

The geriatric social worker will interview patients and relatives on matters regarding the social services, finance and allowances. She will also advise on all statutory and voluntary services.

Attached to the day hospital, either separately or in combination, there will be a technical workshop with a technical instructor in charge. Patients participate in occupations making various aids and articles requiring special movements as part of their rehabilitation.

The majority of patients suffer from a major disability such as locomotor disease, a stroke or various forms of arthritis, but commonly they will have multiple conditions. On first day attendance the patient is assessed, first by clinical examination, then for any medical investigations and treatment required, then for other forms of therapy such as physiotherapy, occupational therapy and speech therapy.

When a patient has reached the stage of maximum benefit resulting in a plateau of functional ability, then consideration must be given to discharge, at either a review clinic or a case conference. Some patients will require further support; they may be introduced to a club or day centre. It is important to hold regular clinics for initial assessment, arranging a programme of therapy, review of progress and final discharge. In this way one can ensure a regular flow of patients through the day hospital, thus creating places for new patients. It has been shown that rehabilitation patients attend for periods of about three months. On the other hand, social patients may attend for a year or more and both they and their relatives becomes very easily dependent on the day hospital. Social intercourse is obviously valuable, particularly for the many patients who live isolated at home, but this should not be the only reason for the patient occupying a place in the day hospital. Attendance at a day centre may be just as helpful.

Figure 5 illustrates where the admissions come from and to where they are eventually discharged.

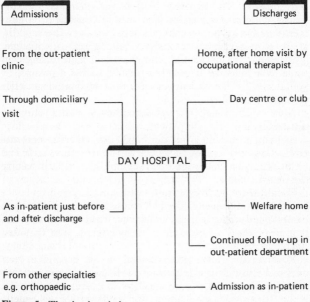

Figure 5. The day hospital.

The patient's day   Before the patient attends the day hospital, he and his relatives will have had clear instructions as to the days he is required to attend, so that he is ready when the ambulance man calls in the morning. The ambulance man can report a patient's difficulty in attending so that this can be quickly investigated by the social worker, health visitor or general practitioner.

The patients arrive in sitting ambulances which may have been collecting several people from a particular area. The ambulance crews should be specially picked for their patience and understanding attitude to elderly people, as not infrequently the patient is not ready or is even still in bed. Incidentally, the ambulance service is the most costly single item in day hospital care. Voluntary car service is also available for ambulant patients, thus relieving the pressure on the ambulance service.

On arrival the patients are greeted by the staff and given refreshments. The morning is spent on individual therapy, clinics, clinical examination and medical treatment. Assessments are carried out on activities of daily living—dressing, the ability to manage lavatory facilities, bathing, self-care, kitchen. Throughout the day baths, chiropody and hairdressing continue. A launderette is usually available, staffed if possible by volunteers, so that patients can get their washing done while visting the hospital.

After lunch, which is a social occasion as well as ensuring satisfactory nutrition, the patients will have a rest. The afternoon is spent on music and group movement, art, entertainment and crafts. Sometimes a church service will be arranged. At the end of the afternoon, following tea, the ambulance will call to take the patients home.

Usually there is a library trolley with special large-print books available. The Women's Royal Voluntary Service trolley shop comes round with toiletries, confectionery and other articles and is a great source of pleasure to many patients who are often unable to get to the shops.

Relatives are encouraged to attend the day hospital at least once to discuss any problems arising at home and to see what the elderly patient is able to do and how to encourage activity at home. If necessary the therapist and social worker will make a home visit to assess special aids and adaptations necessary for the patient to gain as much independence as possible in the community.

Day centres

Day centres are organized and run by voluntary organizations such as Age Concern UK. However, some are run by the social services and some jointly with the district health authority. An innovation is the development of day centres attached to the community hospital. It is important to differentiate between day hospitals and day centres. The latter provide social facilities only and are run by voluntary lay workers with a voluntary nurse in attendance; no specialist medical services are provided and they are not normally attached to hospitals. They are *holding units* rather than therapeutic areas and provide support in the community. However, the elderly person can attend as frequently and for as long as he wishes. Bathing and chiropody services are available, and usually a launderette. Day centres, like day hospitals, provide social contact and distraction for the lonely and housebound. They are suitable for those who require the minimum of supervision. Voluntary transport is essential, for example a minibus, which enables the housebound and the more disabled, who are the people most in need, to attend.

The first aim of those concerned with the welfare of the elderly is to keep them as fit as possible, and since old people need a sense of belonging, enable them to live in their own homes, either alone or with their families. Many are able to continue to lead the kind of life they have always enjoyed, supported by family and friends, and may never require care from health or social services. However, from the age of 80 years onwards, the elderly are more frail and more prone to disease so that there is a greater likelihood that help may be needed.

References

Austin, R. & Parish, P. (1976) Prescribing in general practice. *J. Roy. Coll. Gen. Pract.* Vol. 26 (suppl.) pp. 44–49.

DHSS (1981) *Growing Older*. London: HMSO.

Williamson, J. & Chopin, J.M. (1980) Adverse reactions to prescribed drugs in the elderly. A multicentre investigation. *Age and Ageing* Vol. 9, No. 2.

Further reading

Brocklehurst, J.C. (1970) *The Geriatric Day Hospital*. King Edward's Hospital Fund for London.

Corp, M. & Campbell, J. (1983) *Staying Put*. Anchor Housing Trust. *Help for Older Home Owners*. Age Concern England.

Tinker, A. (1981) *The Elderly in Modern Society*. London: Longman.

3
Care of the Elderly in Hospital: The Geriatric Unit

In order to understand the management of the ill elderly in hospital, the nurse must understand the functions and organization of the geriatric unit. The functions are:

1 To maintain the functional independence—physical, mental and social—of the aged person and so postpone or avoid institutional treatment.
2 To teach.
3 To undertake research.

First, it is essential to have an adequate number of beds for the elderly population in the unit catchment area. The normal yardstick is 10 beds per 1000 but this, of course, will vary according to other facilities in the area such as nursing homes, rest homes and various forms of sheltered housing. Because the number of beds is large, possibly several hundred, widely disseminated throughout the area, and because requests for beds are made from many sources, such as community, rest homes and other hospital departments, it is essential to have a central office with full secretarial staff; this ensures co-ordination and good communication during working hours.

The office and main unit for acute admissions should be sited within a general hospital. This enables the patients to be investigated satisfactorily with facilities for laboratory and radiological investigations. The opinions of consultants in other specialties are more easily obtained.

In-patients

It has been shown from experience that a system of progressive patient care provides the most effective results. The main criticism of this form of care is the sometimes frequent moves for patients, depending on their progress or deterioration. All patients are admitted initially to the *acute assessment and intensive care wards*. In these wards they will be thoroughly examined clinically, mentally and functionally. Routine investigations and any other investigations indicated will be carried out. After a period of 4–6 weeks' treatment a decision will be taken regarding the patient's future. It has been found that approximately a third of the patients will die during this initial period, and a third will recover sufficiently to be discharged back to the community, possibly with more support or supervision than they were receiving prior to admission. The remaining third can be transferred to a *rehabilitation ward*, where the emphasis will be upon regaining personal independence—the ability to wash, visit the lavatory, dress and walk. During this phase of rehabilitation further treatment and nursing will be required. Alternatively, the patient will be moved to a *continuing care* annexe if he is unable to cope with the rehabilitation programme. Here, improvement may take place for up to one year to 18 months later.

When a patient recovers reasonable independence but for various social reasons is unable to return to the community, he will be moved to an *ambulant ward* or '*halfway house*' with a low staff/patient ratio. Ideally a self-care unit or flat should be attached to this ward. Patients may then live independently but under supervision until the social workers have made arrangements for suitable accommodation in the community. This part of the unit is especially useful for patients returning home to live alone.

Some patients cannot respond to treatment or rehabilitation and they may need so much nursing care that they are unable to return to the community under any circumstances. These patients are moved to one of the *continuing care* annexes when a bed is available (see chapter 4). This may be regarded as a medical and/or social failure, but for such patients it is the best place to live.

Specialized wards
In some well established units there will be wards run jointly with other specialties.

Psychogeriatric assessment wards are wards where elderly patients will be seen by the geriatrician, psychiatrist and, if necessary, social worker of the social services department. After a suitable assessment the patient will be transferred either to a geriatric unit ward or to a psychiatric ward for further treatment and care. This arrangement lessens the likelihood of the patient being misplaced and receiving the wrong care, which is to his detriment. Both the acute geriatric and psychiatric beds should be situated in the district general hospitals, thus obviating the need for psychogeriatric assessment wards as liaison and communication between the two would then be greatly improved.

Orthopaedic/geriatric units have been shown to improve the outcome of patients, particularly those with fractured femurs, amputations and following mobilization surgery. The surgery and postoperative care is supervised by the orthopaedic surgeon and his staff, whereas the general care of the patient and his rehabilitation is the responsibility of the geriatric unit. Joint ward rounds are carried out by both consultants.

A *hemiplegic unit* orientated to intensive rehabilitation of 'stroke' patients increases the patient's prospects of maximum recovery.

While working in the geriatric unit the nurse becomes an important member of a large and complex team, as illustrated in Fig. 6.

Admission to hospital

Admission of the elderly patient to hospital is never a very welcome procedure, and the nurse should help to make it as easy and as pleasant as possible. It has often been preceded by a visit by the consultant geriatrician to the patient's home; he will have explained to both the patient and the relatives the reasons for admission and the environment into which the patient will go. The patient is generally acutely ill and requires hospitalization for treatment of this acute illness. Very often the acute illness is superimposed upon a chronic disability. The crisis leading to complete dependency often brings to light an unsuspected semi-dependent state.

One patient admitted to the unit had recently suffered a cerebrovascular accident leaving her with a left hemiplegia. She had been treated during the past years for rheumatoid arthritis, diabetes mellitus, ischaemic heart disease and hypertension; she had come to terms with all these disabilities and was leading a full and independent life, living alone in a bungalow. However, after her cerebrovascular accident she required a period of hospitalization in order to benefit from all the rehabilitation services, and to learn to live with yet another disability.

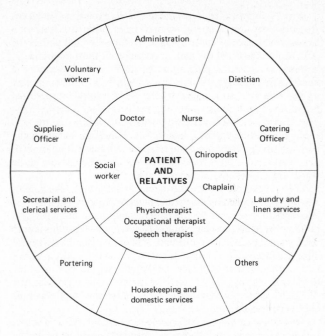

Figure 6. The multidisciplinary team concerned with the care of patients in hospital.

Sometimes the chronic disease has progressed to such a degree that the patient can no longer manage at home. The geriatric unit investigates and treats the patient, then aims towards rehabilitation so that he is fit to return home, where he can live a fuller and more independent life. Whatever support and aids he may need can be organized while he is in hospital.

Occasionally the patient does not respond to treatment as anticipated, or the illness has progressed so that he is unable to respond and may require permanent hospitalization. Holiday beds are available in most units to give relatives a chance to rest and perhaps take a holiday. Some units arrange intermittent admissions to help the relatives cope with severe disability. Some beds are used on a monthly basis so that two patients use the same bed on alternate months. This can be successful once the patient has become used to the idea and to the staff.

Loss of independence, a change of surroundings and confrontation by innumerable strange faces often precipitates a temporary degree of confusion and even resentment within the patient. Reception of the patient on arrival is most important in helping to create the right atmosphere from the beginning: a cheerful welcome from the staff, after which he is shown quietly to his own bed and locker where he can store his personal possessions, and given a cup of tea or coffee. The welcome extended has a great bearing on the patient's ability to settle into the ward routine and will also have a beneficial effect on the co-operation received from the relatives. All these things help to allay the patient's fear. He should also be shown the layout of the ward and the toilet facilities available.

The nurses' approach to the patient is important. The patient should be addressed by his correct name and not by some term of endearment except where the patient requests to be called by a familiar pet name, and care should be taken to see that this is only used when specifically requested. The name should always be clearly written above the bed for all to see. When addressing the patient the nurse should face the patient and talk to him at his level, so that he can see the nurse's expression and lip movement; the nurse must not stand over him, addressing him above or behind his head.

One lady aged 98 years, admitted from an old people's home, was quite amazed to find she had come into hospital when she saw all the empty beds, as she had no idea that patients were not confined to their beds while receiving treatment!

When the nurse has seen the patient comfortably installed, and introduced him to the patient in the next bed, his suitcase is unpacked and all his belongings placed in his locker. At the same time the nurse can see if he has any valuable articles with him. Many elderly people bring all their worldly goods with them, including large sums of money and valuable jewellery. With the patient's consent these should be either sent home with the relatives or locked away in the hospital safe. The hospital authorities are not responsible for the patient's property. If he insists on keeping it, this should be made clear to him at the time.

Relatives

Relatives often accompany the patient into hospital and they too should be given a warm and friendly welcome. Their help and co-operation will be needed during the patient's stay, and therefore their reception is of great importance. They are often upset at their mother or father being admitted to a geriatric unit rather than the medical ward, and if the nurse explains the work of the unit at the beginning, resentment and fears can be allayed.

Accurate information can be obtained from the relatives as to the patient's age, address, family doctor and other particulars. Ideally the unit should arrange open visiting hours, so that relatives and friends can come and go at their own convenience. The nurse should try to encourage the relatives to visit at hours when they can help with some of the patient's care, such as feeding, bathing or walking.

Often relatives are frightened by the hospital atmosphere and the bustle of the staff, and no longer feel competent to do what they have been doing so admirably at home. Some also feel they have done enough and are relieved to sit back and have a rest. One devoted daughter, who had looked after a rather trying mother and was really in need of a rest, insisted on visiting twelve hours a day and greatly impeded her mother's progress, despite tactful remarks from the nursing staff, social workers and the general practitioner.

The nursing process

The nursing process has been introduced as a vehicle for improving the quality of nursing care. It has four main elements—assessment, planning, implementation and evaluation. The philosophy of patient care involves trying to improve the quality of life for the patient so that he can realize his full potential as a human being. This involves not only providing the basic needs of food, shelter and sleep, but also helping him to achieve the greatest degree of mobility and independence in daily living with as much aid as he requires. In order to achieve this satisfactorily, the nurse will find the implementation of an individualized care plan a great asset. In order to devise this, a nursing history is first taken and from this the nurse can learn about the personality of the patient and his life-style, and so help to preserve his identity and sustain his morale. A care plan can then be devised tailor-made to the patient and altered as necessary (see Fig. 7). An evaluation should be made at regular intervals so that the nursing and therapeutic team can determine whether progress is being made, or if the goals are set too high

Figure 7. A sample care plan.

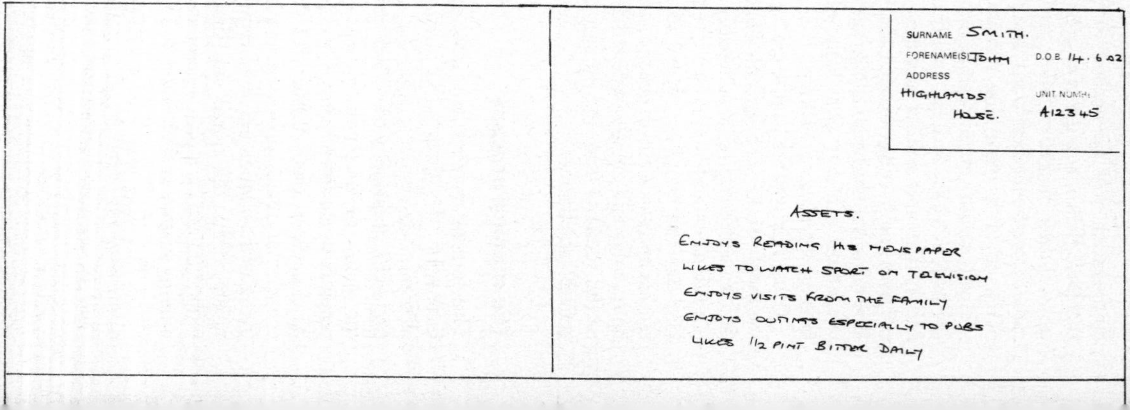

SURNAME _SMITH._
FORENAME(S) [ ] BIM   D.O.B. 14. 6. 02
ADDRESS   UNIT NUMBER
HIGHLANDS   A·23·45
      HOSP.

ASSETS.

ENJOYS READING THE NEWSPAPER

LIKES TO WATCH SPORT ON TELEVISION

ENJOYS VISITS FROM THE FAMILY

GENERALLY OUTINGS ESPECIALLY TO PUBS

LIKES 1/2 PINT BITTER DAILY

DIAGNOSIS: CEREBRO/VASCULAR ACCIDENT. LEFT HEMI PLEGIA AGE 81

Date	No	Problem Need	Aim of Care	Date	No	Care Required	Signature	Date Resolved/ Changed Signature
8.1.84	1.	TENDENCY TO INCONTINENCE DUE TO IMMOBILITY	1. TO MAINTAIN CONTINENCE		1.	HELP TO LAVATORY 2 HOURLY. VARIED OPENING TO TROUSERS. URINAL BY SIDE AT NIGHT.	A Brown	
	2.	CONSTIPATION	2. TO PREVENT		2a.	ENCOURAGE FLUIDS AND DIET & BRAN.	A Brown	
					b	ROUGHAGE AT NIGHT.		
	3.	DIFFICULTY WASHING	3. TO HELP AS NECESSARY		3.	6-7DAYS DAILY BATH AT NIGHT. HELP WITH WASHING IN THE MORNING.	A Brown	
	4.	NIGHT COUGH	4. TO RELIEVE.		4.	SETTLE WITH WARM DRINK. LINCTUS IF REQUIRED.	A Brown	
	5.	LEFT SIDED WEAKNESS	5. TO HAVE PHYSIO THERAPY AND OCCUPATIONAL THERAPY TO IMPROVE MOBILITY		5.	DAILY ATTENDANCE IN DEPARTMENT.	K	

Date	Nos. of Care Given	Nursing Report Evaluation of Progress	Signature	Date	Evaluation	Signature
18.1.84	1	Managing well	R	25.1.84	Has regood work, managed to maintain	R
	2.	Bowels well open.	⌐		Continence with help, employed a ball	
	3.	Engaged & such.	⌐		Bath night. C cough has improved, enjoyed	Roberts
					A trip to the Pub. Has attended physiotherapy	
					and occupational therapy daily. Mobis	
					improving, can almost belts un-aided.	

and need to be altered. The nursing history should cover all aspects of the patient's life-style, so that the nurse has a true picture of the patient. She should discover where he lives and in what surroundings, and who supports him at home. She should also investigate his sleep pattern, his dietary requirements, his bowel and bladder function and all other aspects—including his interests, hobbies and pets. In order to obtain a clear picture, the history is necessarily long and detailed, and in order not to tire the patient, it might be wise for the nurse to cover it in several sessions. From the history any problems can be highlighted and listed, but for the elderly it is essential that the nurse does not dwell unduly on problems and highlights assets as well—these can be assessed when the history is being taken.

Having listed the problems, the care plan can be devised with the care required for each problem and an evaluation made at suitable intervals to ensure that progress is being made and that goals are being attained. By adopting this kind of philosophy the nurse should be able to ensure that the patient's personality is not weakened in a new environment, that he retains his self-esteem, and that there is minimal regimentation and institutionalization.

Routine observations

Weight   On admission the patient should be weighed routinely and subsequently weekly during his stay in the acute hospital ward, as weight gains and losses are important and have a direct bearing on his diagnosis and future treatment. In some instances, e.g. gross heart failure, where large doses of diuretics are given, it may be necessary to weigh the patient daily to test the efficiency of the drugs.

Urine   Urine should be tested on the patient's admission for acidity, specific gravity, sugar, acetone, albumen, blood and bile. The use of Bili-labstix makes all this a quick and simple procedure. Many elderly diabetics, who have remained undiagnosed until admission, have been detected in this way. A clean specimen of urine should be sent to the laboratory for analysis as urinary tract infections are common in old age.

Temperature, pulse and respiration   In assessment and rehabilitation wards it is often expedient to observe the patient's temperature, pulse and respiration rate daily for a short period after admission, as deviation from the normal may be the first sign that all is not well. However, the nurse should not become obsessed with these observations to the detriment of other more important caring roles.

Blood pressure   Blood pressure may be recorded daily for one week unless otherwise requested by the doctor so that a clear pattern of blood pressure can be charted. It must be remembered that patients suffering from giddiness and falls should have their blood pressure recorded both lying and standing in order to eliminate postural hypotension. Those who suffer from high or low blood pressure or who are taking tablets to control blood pressure will obviously have their blood pressure recorded more frequently and for a longer period of time.

Bowel function   Daily recording of bowel function is important and aperients should be administered in the evening if necessary. Use of the patient's regular aperient may often allay anxiety over the precipitant bowel action, but Dorbanex suspension, Mil-Par, Duphalac and Senokot amongst others have proved to have a gentle and efficient action. Administration of glycerol or bisacodyl suppositories may relieve discomfort following absence of bowel action for 2 or 3 days, but an enema saponis is usually no more uncomfortable and has a more efficient action. There are a variety of proprietary brands of enema on the market, mainly of the disposable type, but they do not appear to be as efficient as soap and water.

General nursing care

Bathing the patient in the bathroom
Many elderly may not have had a bath for years and may be very apprehensive at doing so. The nurse should be very reassuring and not force any patient to bath unless he wants to. The bathroom should be warm and the nurse should take care that the patient does not feel the cold. The patient may be bathed with use of the Ambulift, in an ordinary bath with aids, in a Medic bath, or in a Parker bath.

If the Ambulift is used the patient may be wheeled to the bathroom on the chair if necessary. Either the chair lift or slings may be used for bathing. If the former is used, its arms can be removed to allow free movement once the patient is seated safely in the bath. The water should be kept at approximately 38°C and plenty of water run in so that the patient can have a good soak.

If the patient is mobile and able to help himself he may be able to manage a bath without any mechanical aid. A non-slip bath mat, bath rails and if necessary a bath seat are all valuable additions. The Medic bath is a sitting bath with a removable front panel, so that the patient can step into the bath only over a low step. It is used in conjunction with a shower. The Ladywell Bath System is designed for severely handicapped people, who are wheeled into the bath on a specially designed chair; the end of the bath is then closed, and the bath filled. The Parker bath opens at the side and the patient can slide across on to the seat from a wheelchair. Water can be run into the base before the patient enters, and the bath can be tilted so the patient can relax and soak in warm surroundings. Towels and clean clothing should be made available before the bath is begun so that the patient is not kept waiting. Bathing is often a good opportunity for the nurse to have an uninterrupted talk with the patient.

Showering the patient
Showers are also very useful and refreshing. The elderly patient often seems alarmed at the idea, but once having had one nearly always seems to enjoy them thoroughly. It is essential that the shower room is very warm. Clean towels and fresh clothing should all be prepared beforehand. The nurse should make herself familiar with the thermostat, so that the shower water is neither too hot nor too cold. The patient can be rinsed all over, washed with a soapy flannel and then thoroughly rinsed again. Often the patient is able to operate the shower spray himself and only needs assistance with his back and sacrum. The shower is very useful for incontinent patients as the nurse is able to clean the sacral area with ease.

Pressure areas
Pressure areas should be treated 2–4 hourly, depending on the condition and mobility of the patient, and his position changed as necessary. This subject is discussed in more detail in chapter 7.

Dental care and oral hygiene

Food is one of the essential physical needs of the elderly. Enjoyment of food is dependent on dental comfort, and it is very important that proper attention is paid to mouth and dental hygiene.

Decaying teeth are often seen in the elderly and referral should be made to a dentist if necessary. Ill-fitting dentures may also be remedied while in hospital. These should be identified with a denture marker to prevent loss. Patients often arrive without their dentures, which they have not worn for years, due to a fault or discomfort. Some small faults may be easily corrected if they are brought into hospital.

Teeth, false or natural, should be cleaned every morning and/or evening. If the patient is unable to do this for himself, the nurse should do so, soaking false teeth as necessary in a specific denture cleaner. Many elderly people prefer not to be seen without false teeth and usually replace them for the night, after cleaning. In the case of natural teeth, the nurse should ensure that the patient has his own toothbrush and toothpaste, and assist with cleaning if necessary.

For the very sick patient oral toilet should be performed 2–4 hourly. A tray for this purpose should be set daily, and not left by the bedside to accumulate dust.

The most effective method of cleaning the mouth of the patient who is unable to help himself is by using a disposable glove, with a piece of gauze wrapped round the finger and dipped in a solution of thymol compound. Artery forceps wrapped with gauze may also be used, as may a disposable toothbrush. Orange sticks must not be used for this purpose as they are dangerous and can penetrate the gums.

A very dirty mouth may benefit from being cleaned with a solution of one part hydrogen peroxide to three parts warm water. Monilia infection occurring in the mouth must be treated with a course of nystatin or amphotericin. Finally the mouth can be swabbed with glycerine to encourage salivary secretion. Dry lips can be moistened with petroleum jelly or white Vaseline. The nurse must be aware of drugs and food particles collecting in the corners of the mouth; these can lead to ulceration and infection. When this is liable to occur, the mouth should be well cleaned after every meal. It is also important to encourage frequent drinks, as some elderly are loath to take fluids even when they are able and a drink is available.

Care of nails and feet

Nails benefit from a manicure, especially toe-nails, which may have been totally neglected. The Red Cross run a short course in manicure and volunteers from this course are particularly useful and welcome in the geriatric unit. A visiting chiropodist is an asset to treat onychogryphosis (overgrown, horny toe-nails), hallux valgus (bunions) and corns, all of which result in the patient wearing ill-fitting footwear, leading to difficulty in walking. These conditions may also be the cause of falls in the elderly. The feet of elderly diabetic patients need particular attention.

Mrs X., a retired nurse aged 81 years, was referred to the geriatrician with several problems, including intermittent attacks of gastroenteritis, and having become chair-fast she was doubly incontinent and depressed. She was found to have severe onychogryphosis with ulceration, and once this had been dealt with by the chiropodist, she again became fully ambulant, no longer incontinent and able to return home to her husband.

Care of hair

A geriatric unit should view the patient as a whole and not just consider his acute illness. Thus a visit to the unit is a good time to remedy some of the smaller problems also. A haircut and shampoo are often appreciated by those living alone and quite frequently cases of seborrhoea can be treated with medicated shampoos such as Sebbix and severe cases with selenium sulphide. It is usually unnecessary to wash the hair in bed, and this can be done in the bath or shower room. Most units have a hairdresser who visits weekly, and the renewal of a permanent wave or set will often do much to boost the patient's morale.

Deafness and hearing-aids

Difficulty in hearing has often been accepted as a hazard of old age for which there is no remedy, although in many cases the ears are filled with wax and benefit from being syringed. Olive oil drops for two days before treatment are a help when syringing is needed or a wax softener, such as Cerumol, can be used.

Some patients may need a hearing-aid and can be referred to the ear, nose and throat department while in hospital. Those who already have an aid often need assistance as well. Some may have difficulty penetrating the wax. One elderly nun was convinced her aid was no good, yet when she removed the ear-piece it was completely blocked with wax. Even porridge has been discovered there!

While the patient is in hospital it is often a good time for the hearing aid to be overhauled by the audiometrician. Broken parts can be replaced and new batteries can be supplied. New ear moulds can be taken if needed and new pieces fitted. Batteries should be changed every 2–4 weeks and a good supply should be readily available. The irritating whistle of hearing-aids is caused by the amplifier being too near the receiver or by an ill-fitting ear-piece. The introduction by the National Health Service of the behind-the-ear aid has eliminated some of the problems, but each individual needs to be assessed according to his special needs.

One must remember that a hearing-aid does not improve intelligibility of speech and one must still speak clearly and slowly. When speaking to a hard-of-hearing person, emphasis must be placed on the consonant and not on the vowel. When saying 'bread and butter' emphasize BR--D -ND B-TT-R, not --EA- A-- -U--E-. If the patient has just acquired a new aid, great patience must be exercised and encouragement given to him to use it. Initial use is very tiring and should only be for short periods of time in a quiet place, as background noises are also amplified and can be very distressing. The Department of Health and Social Security have issued a booklet *General Guidance for Hearing Aid Users* which is given to all receivers of new aids and contains a lot of useful information.

Sight and spectacles

Spectacles may need to be checked and a visit to the optician can usually be arranged. These also should be inconspicuously identified with the patient's name on admission, as they can be easily mislaid and not every owner can recognize his own glasses. The ophthalmologist is always available to see patients with abnormalities of vision and advise them what needs to be done.

Lifting

Much of the nurse's time within the geriatric unit is spent lifting, and it is essential that she is taught to do this correctly so that she does not suffer any injury to herself. Elderly people and especially hemiplegic patients are not always able to co-operate fully owing to their disabilities and therefore orthodox lifts are not always used. These basic points should be followed when lifting (see Figs. 8–10):

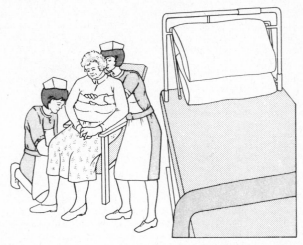

Figure 8. Correct method of lifting an elderly patient from a chair.

1 The nurse should ensure that there is plenty of room to manoeuvre and that all unnecessary equipment is removed so that there are no hazards to fall over.
2 The procedure is explained to the patient and the bedclothes are folded back.
3 The two lifters, ideally, should be of approximately the same height and should decide which type of lift they are going to use.
4 The nurse should adopt the correct posture: the back should be straight, the knees and hips bent, the thigh and hip muscles being used to straighten the legs and thus lift the patient. The feet should be far enough apart to allow for an even distribution of weight. The lifters must work together.
5 On completion of the lift, the bedclothes should be replaced and the patient settled comfortably.

Clothing
Patients feel more at home wearing their own clothes wherever possible, and once they are over their acute illness they are encouraged to be up and dressed. Particular importance is laid

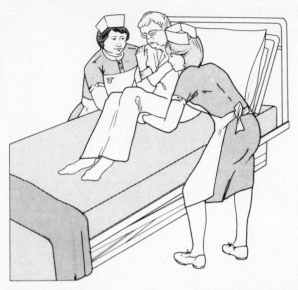

Figure 9. Correct method of lifting an elderly patient up the bed.

upon shoes, which should provide good support and comfort. If possible shoes rather than slippers should be worn, although it is often quite a battle to convert some patients to wearing shoes after years of only ever wearing slippers. An arrangement with the local shoe shop is often helpful when fitting the patient with new shoes. All clothes and shoes should be marked on arrival, as has already been mentioned for false teeth, spectacles and hearing-aids, as it is amazing how quickly articles (especially underwear) disappear.

Drug administration

Drugs are administered at regular intervals throughout the day in accordance with the written instructions of the doctor. Each patient will be following his individual regimen.

Diuretics should always be given early in the day, so that they do not interfere with the patient's rest at night. The nurse should check that the patient has actually swallowed the tablets—so often one finds small bundles hidden in a handkerchief or under

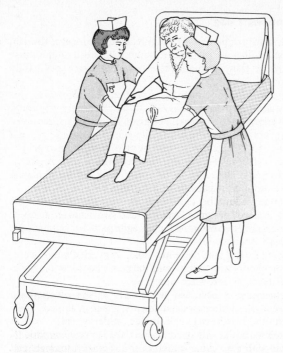

Figure 10. Correct method of lifting an elderly patient up the bed, holding the patient's arms.

the pillows even though the patient was seen to put them in his mouth.

A simple explanation of the action of the tablets often helps, as the patient can see the reason for their administration. One should always, if possible, let the patient take the tablet himself, rather than thrusting it directly into his mouth, which is most unpleasant. Some tablets are large and difficult to swallow; if necessary they can usually be replaced by a suspension, or a soluble tablet. Injections are often unavoidable, and the sites should be rotated so that the patient does not become sore in one spot.

The patient's day

As the majority of patients in the unit are up for most of the day, it should be planned for their maximum comfort, so the nurse must ensure they have adequate rest, but also remain fully occupied.

It is general for patients to be up for breakfast. However, this does not mean that patients have to be woken excessively early. An early morning cup of tea can be given before the patient rises. It is not easy for even the most agile person to eat in bed, and impossible for the hemiplegic or otherwise incapacitated patient to do so with ease and comfort. Patients enjoy their meals far more sitting in a chair, and at the same time it eliminates having to feed a number of patients individually.

Everyone should be aided and encouraged to go to the lavatory, and well designed lavatories and sanichairs are an asset. Commodes are often essential for less agile patients, but bedpans rarely need be used.

Dressing should take place in a calm, unhurried atmosphere, as independently as possible, and the staff should be taught to give assistance as and when necessary.

The morning is occupied with visits to the occupational therapy and physiotherapy departments, a bath or shower, and a visit from the hairdresser, chiropodist or clergyman.

The nurse should aim at a daily bath for incontinent patients and those with indwelling catheters or a vaginal discharge, and every other day for the rest of the patients. Many have not had a bath for several years, and do not relish the idea when in hospital, but after the first visit are nearly always pleased to go again. The Ambulift has proved invaluable for the nurse and provides a comfortable, safe method of moving the patient in and out of the bath.

Lunch served at a communal table can be enjoyed by many, after which some patients like to have an hour's rest on their bed or in a comfortable chair. We have found the Buxton chair ideal for those patients who tend to slide forward out of the ordinary upright varieties; the tipping device prevents slide and enables the patient to have a peaceful rest. The nurse must remember to support the legs and feet of the patient, thus preventing pressure on the back of the thighs. An hour in the afternoon may be devoted to some form of group activity, such as bingo, a whist drive, music and movement, painting or the showing of slides.

The nursing staff usually take it in turn to organize this and it proves a challenge both for them and for the patients. Voluntary workers can be successfully incorporated into these activities too.

Most patients wash their hands and face after tea and are then encouraged to get undressed and retire to bed after supper. By this time they are usually quite tired and ready for a good night's rest, often without the aid of any sedation. Should sedatives be necessary, barbiturates should be avoided, and if possible temazepam or Heminevrin used instead. Barbiturates tend to increase rather than reduce the patient's disorientation and restlessness. It is important that noise, both human and mechanical, is reduced to the minimum.

Care of the unconscious patient

During her time in the geriatric unit the nurse will come in contact with the unconscious patient and must be aware of the principles involved in caring for this patient.

The most common cause of unconsciousness in the elderly is a cerebrovascular accident due to thrombosis, embolus or haemorrhage. It may occasionally be due to poisoning by gas, drugs or alcohol. Infection may be the cause with resulting septicaemia, encephalitis or meningitis. Other causes include severe myxoedema, diabetes, uraemia, hypothermia, hyperthermia, dehydration and cerebral tumours.

On admission the observations which the doctor will ask the nurse to record will vary according to the cause of unconsciousness. In all cases a record of temperature, pulse, respiration and blood pressure will be required at frequent intervals.

The patient will be nursed on his side, the elderly patient usually being nursed in the lateral position, occasionally in the semi-prone position. He must be well supported so that he cannot roll on to his back causing obstruction of the airway with possible inhalation of secretions. It will be necessary to have near at hand:

- Oxygen cylinder and face mask
- Suction apparatus
- Rubber airway
- Mouth gag
- Tongue-holding forceps
- Tongue depressor

It is most important that the nurse maintain a clear airway at all times by keeping the nostrils clear, removing any false teeth and using the suction apparatus to remove any secretions, sputum or vomit.

The patient should have his position changed 2-hourly, both day and night. As elderly people are particularly prone to pressure sores, it is usually wise to nurse the unconscious patient on a ripple bed or some other pressure-relieving mattress from the outset. This, however, does not lessen the need for regular turning by the nurse. Regular turning also helps to lessen the risk of chest complications and enables the nurse or physiotherapist to perform passive movements on all the limbs, thus reducing the risk of contractures. When the patient is at rest, the limbs should be well supported on pillows or foam pads, to prevent areas of skin touching each other.

The nurse will wash the patient regularly, taking special care to dry under the folds of the breasts and in the groins. The mouth will be cleaned regularly and the lips kept moist. The eyes should be bathed routinely with a solution of half-strength normal saline, and kept free from crusts.

As the patient is incontinent, catheterization is usually recommended, unless the patient appears to be regaining consciousness quickly. Regular bowel habit should be encouraged by insertion of glycerol suppositories, or by digital removal of faeces by an experienced nurse. After a few days a regular pattern may evolve without the aid of medication.

Initially the unconscious patient will be given intravenous fluids, the quantity and quality determined by the doctor, depending on the electrolyte balance and the cause of unconsciousness. If there is no rapid improvement in the level of unconsciousness, it is normal to progress to nasogastric feeding, as this provides an easier method for regulating the nutritional intake of the patient. The type of feeds given will be discussed by the doctor, nurse and dietitian, depending on the patient's needs (see chapter 8).

Nursing the unconscious patient demands skill and patience on the part of the nurse. She must remember that the patient is still an individual even though he may be unable to communicate and the nurse should never discuss his condition or his affairs at the bedside.

Preparation for discharge

The aim of the geriatric unit is to make the patient fit and ready for discharge due to successful treatment and rehabilitation. As always, the whole team is involved, including all those in the community, as careful preparation for discharge is always required. A suitable day will be selected well in advance and the relatives or friends informed. Transport will be ordered; the general practitioner, health visitor and community nurse will all be informed in good time. The check-list on the nursing care plan will ensure that all arrangements are made and drugs ordered if necessary.

Discharge is frequently preceded by a home visit from the occupational therapist, physiotherapist and/or social worker, accompanied by the patient, to see what problems exist at home. A relative or friend should also be present to give some help and learn what has been decided. It is helpful if the community nurse is also present, as she can discuss the problems that arose before, and see what has been achieved since, admission to hospital. The visitor will pay particular attention to the layout of the flat or house—whether it is all on the same level or has difficult occasional steps. She will examine the condition of the stairs—whether they are steep; if they have a handrail; whether they are properly lit; and whether the stair carpet is worn or frayed. Any loose mats at the top or bottom should be removed. If the patient is unable to go up and down stairs, she will investigate the possibility of bringing the bed downstairs. Many elderly people do not like sleeping downstairs and will be reluctant to agree to this.

The kitchen should also be looked over closely, and the safety of the cooking equipment checked. However, it is no use changing to a more modern appliance if the patient cannot understand its working and has, over many years, become accustomed to using an ancient cooker. If possible, the oven should be table height to avoid the patient needing to bend over, and possibly dropping hot dishes and getting burnt.

The height of the bed and chair will be noted. The bath too will be inspected; bathing may often prove impossible if the patient lives alone but often it will be found that a special bath seat, bath rails and a non-slip mat on the floor of the bath will enable the patient to manage alone. The lavatory may require appropriate handrails and the seat may need raising. In many cases there may still be only an outside lavatory and a commode may be needed.

Attention will also be paid to the heating appliances—they should be sufficient in number and adequately guarded. Many old people still use paraffin heaters as they are an economical form of heating, but they are potentially dangerous. They should be placed in a safe position where they cannot be knocked over and are free from draughts.

Patients who are to live alone after discharge will have been assessed by the occupational therapist on their ability to dress themselves, to cook for themselves, bath, do their washing and all household chores. The patient may be taken to visit the home prior to discharge so that the therapist and social worker may see how the patient reacts and copes with things in his own environment. This is specially useful in the case of the patient who lives alone and who does not wish to leave the sheltered and supportive atmosphere of the hospital. Once the patient sees his own home again, some enthusiasm returns. On these visits it may be useful for the home nurse or health visitor to be present.

Discharge will never be arranged for a Friday or weekend unless the relatives particularly request it. With few services available over the weekend, it may be disastrous for an elderly person returning to live alone after a spell in hospital to be abandoned for 2 days with no social services.

A home help and meals-on-wheels may have been laid on, depending on the patient's ability and wishes. Many people like to have them until they find their feet again at home. The community nurse may be asked to call to help with bathing or even dressing, and sometimes to dress an ulcer or give an injection. The health visitor may also be requested to visit to assess whether the patient is managing satisfactorily and to ensure that he is continuing to be mobile and active. Often there is no incentive to be mobile at home and relatives and neighbours are too kind and do too much, leaving the patient to sink back into the condition that existed before treatment.

The community liaison nurse will also be involved in preparations for the patient's discharge. She will have met the patient while he was in hospital, assessed the problems and discussed them with the community nurse. In some hospitals she transmits a form containing all relevant details from the ward sister to the home nurse and vice versa. She may also continue to visit the patient at home if there is some particular problem which needs assessment and supervision.

Mrs X., aged 88 years, lived with a truly devoted husband in a pleasant terraced cottage in the country. She was obese and had gradually become less mobile due to osteoarthritis, and incontinence had resulted. The geriatrician visited her and decided that a spell in hospital with intensive rehabilitation was the only possible solution. Progress was slow, impeded by the zealous husband who listened to and sympathized with both parties in the problem, but was always won over by his wife's tears! However, quite good progress was noted and she was eventually discharged home to attend the day hospital regularly to ensure that progress was maintained. However, once she was home, nothing could persuade her to return!

Further reading

Garrett, G. (1983) *Health Needs of the Elderly*. Basingstoke: Macmillan.
Irvine, R.E., Bagnall, M.K. & Smith, B.J. (1978) *The Older Patient*. London: English Universities Press.
Isaacs, B., Burns, E.M. & Gracie, T. (1973) *Geriatric Nursing*. London: Heinemann Medical.
Kratz, C.R. (1979) *The Nursing Process*. London: Baillière Tindall.
Long, R. (1981) *Systematic Nursing Care*. London: Faber & Faber.
Wells, T.J. (1980) *Problems in Geriatric Nursing Care*. New York: Churchill Livingstone.

4
Continuing Care of the Elderly

Those elderly patients who have been admitted to the acute assessment and rehabilitation wards of the geriatric unit and fail to respond sufficiently to their treatment to enable them to return to their own home, warden-controlled flat or residential home, and who require constant nursing care, may need long-term care within the auspices of the geriatric unit. Most of their medical care will have been organized, and physiotherapy and occupational therapy will have been given so that the patients have reached their maximum ability, but they will still need nursing care. These frail elderly may well find themselves on the continuing care or long-stay wards of the geriatric unit. Approximately one third of the elderly entering a geriatric unit may need this type of care.

Some elderly fail to respond to the activity and hard work of the acute unit, but may improve radically in the relaxed atmosphere of a continuing care unit. These few patients may eventually be discharged home into the community.

Accommodation

The siting of these wards is important and not always ideal. Many long-stay units are found in old workhouses, often in an isolated part of the town and in rather dreary surroundings. The elderly still remember the time when old people were taken into custodial care in overcrowded and spartan conditions. These elderly people manage best in small units near their own homes so they can still remain part of the community and be visited frequently by family and friends. As this may be the patient's home for some years, the average length of stay in some units being 1–2 years and in others as long as 5 years, the environment needs to be imaginative with pleasant gardens and grounds where possible. It is also therapeutic for patients to see some activity in the outside world, such as traffic and people passing by, as they should not feel isolated from the community. As this is to be the elderly person's home, it may in fact be more appropriate to refer to the patient as a 'resident', and this will be done for the rest of this chapter.

The rooms need to be bright with colourful curtains and bedspreads, carpets in all areas if possible, plenty of pictures and as many of the resident's personal possessions as space and the fire regulations permit. Adequate day space should be provided so that where possible the residents can eat and socialize away from the bed areas. This is often very difficult to achieve! If possible the elderly who have to enter these units should have a chance to visit first, and see where they are eventually going to live, meeting the staff and all who work there. This gives the staff too the opportunity to discuss life within the ward and the possibility of the resident bringing his own possessions, pictures, ornaments and even a favourite chair with him. Many elderly entering these wards tend to lose their identity and individuality and become one of a group, so every opportunity should be taken by the staff to investigate their past and regard them as individuals with their own likes and dislikes. They should be introduced to other residents of similar interests with whom friendships may be formed, but their individual wishes should be adhered to wherever possible.

Institutionalization

The problem of any group of elderly people living together in an institution is that they may become depersonalized due to their environment and life-style. It is therefore essential that the resident's privacy is respected and personal possessions are encouraged as far as possible. This is often very difficult to achieve in some continuing care units at present. It is necessary that each resident be treated as an individual and not as one of a group. Although in any institution it is politic to have a few rules and regulations, it is also essential that residents have freedom of choice in all matters regarding their life-style. Social integration with their environment and the outside world as well as with the staff all help to reduce the incidence of institutionalization.

Staffing

Nursing within these units is of a specialized nature and not suitable for all nurses. Some prefer to nurse patients where more positive treatment is possible and there is a much quicker turnover of patients within the ward; others feel they have something to offer in this field and enjoy the constant contact with the same residents. Nurses working within these units have to learn to adapt their thinking so that the residents' nursing needs are geared around their social needs and not vice versa. So often nursing routines are allowed to dominate the life of these wards and little time is left for 'living'. Nurses need to be able to combine basic nursing skills with imagination, enthusiasm and a sense of humour and commitment.

Many units are staffed by qualified and unqualified staff only, but there is an important role for the learners who need to learn how to care for the elderly in such settings. How this is incorporated into their training varies with different training schools. Nursing auxiliaries working in this area need a special period of training in how to care for elderly residents in a more home-like environment. It is so important that all staff working in this field understand the needs of the elderly residents, the importance of freedom of choice and the necessity of adapting individual care programmes to that particular resident's needs, not emphasizing the resident's problems but highlighting his assets. It is extremely important to maintain a high morale among the staff and this can only be done by developing a good team spirit, so that all are working together and helping to overcome the many problems and difficulties encountered daily, and enjoying the achievements and activities of these residents. Not only must the nursing staff form a team, but doctors, physiotherapists, occupational therapists, social workers, voluntary workers and relatives must also be encouraged to give their help and support.

Daily life

The nurse should try to investigate the resident's past, his previous occupation, and what happened to his family, so that she can visualize the resident as he was when he was fit and well, and also show a constructive interest in the resident's present affairs. Perhaps the resident has some interesting hobbies and these could be renewed and pursued in hospital. It is surprising how many residents can still perform simple jobs and make themselves useful despite a physical or mental handicap. It is also very important to maintain their self-respect and, if possible, make the residents feel they are useful and have a purpose in life.

The residents should be dressed every day, whenever possible, and should wear their own clothes. Many residents have no suitable clothes and it may be necessary to acquire some for them. Many residents may be able to visit the local shops, and choose and buy their own clothes. Many shops now have good facilities for the disabled. There are easily laundered fabrics available these days at reasonable prices and there is no excuse for an old lady to wear a deceased person's ill-fitting cast-offs. Wearing their own clothes gives residents an identity and pride in their appearance. They should also be encouraged to wear good shoes; no one can attempt to walk successfully if they only wear bedroom slippers, giving no support to the feet. Specially adapted clothing for the severely disabled is now readily available and can usually be acquired on contract through the hospital suppliers. There are a variety of attractively designed and coloured dresses specifically for the disabled and incontinent. For ladies there are short vests, split dresses and skirts in synthetic materials, which are easily washable and require little or no ironing. Self-support hose remove the necessity for corsets and suspender belts. Of course, pants should be worn at all times. For the men there are specially adapted trousers with Velcro fastenings and openings as necessary. There are also specially adapted braces and toe-less socks, sweaters of various descriptions and coats split down the middle with a Velcro fastening for the immobile patient. For the bedridden there are now a variety of night-dresses which are easy to put on, but do not have an institutional look. Laundering of the residents' own clothing often proves difficult. Ideally, but not often practically, it is best if the visitors can assist in this field. In many units a launderette has now been installed so that a personalized clothing system is in operation. All clothing is individually labelled and laundered on site, the residents having their own laundry bags, so that loss and damage to garments is reduced to a minimum. Although marking poses a problem, it is essential, and no system entirely satisfactory. It is, however, a job that can be undertaken by visitors or voluntary workers.

Incontinence is also a problem often encountered in the continuing care unit and must be treated optimistically with a realistic outlook by the staff. If all other methods fail, there should be no reservations in resorting to a catheter and leg bag during the day and free drainage at night. It is also possible to have the tubing of the catheter bag passing through the vest seam and the bag itself contained in a sponge bag. This is more satisfactory than a spigot when the resident is up, as the latter tends to cause more frequent urinary tract infection. Faecal incontinence should rarely occur if the resident's bowel habits are well supervised. Incontinence is discussed in detail in chapter 6.

The residents must be encouraged to maintain a pride in their appearance, and a regular visit from a hairdresser is a necessity. Nothing is more successful in boosting the morale of the elderly lady than to have her hair permed or set. Similarly the elderly men should have a daily shave and a visit from the barber when necessary. Nails should be kept clean and short. Hearing-aids should be kept in good working order, and false teeth should be seen to be comfortable and well-fitting.

Feeding, too, may prove a problem. The residents should be encouraged to feed themselves for as long as possible. It can be most degrading and unpleasant being fed by someone else. In

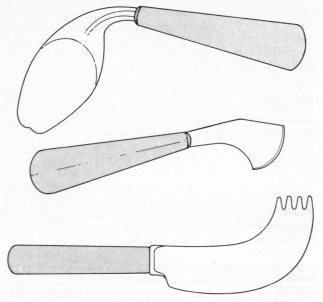

Figure 11. Feeding aids: a Manoy spoon, a Manoy knife and a Nelson knife.

order to feed himself easily and successfully the resident should be sitting as comfortably as possible, preferably in a chair, as it is difficult to sit upright in bed, with easy access to the table and tray. Various aids should be available on the ward to help residents with specific disabilities. Hemiplegic patients have difficulty in managing single-handed and may benefit from a plate bunker or bowl produced by Melaware products especially designed for the handicapped and disabled. The Nelson knife may be beneficial in certain cases. Melaware, in their Manoy range of goods, also produce a well-designed cup and various pieces of cutlery which may be of help to those disabled by arthritis or who have Parkinson's disease. These three diseases especially provide many problems for the staff and at mealtimes. A table napkin should be provided at all times to avoid undue soiling of clothing. Presentation of food is also important and some handicapped residents find food that can be eaten with the fingers easier to manage. Mealtimes should be social events with everyone eating in the day area where possible. In many units a menu service is now available with a choice of different dishes at each meal. This choice should be made as near to the meal as possible. In smaller units the cook may get to know the residents quite well and be able to cater for many of their specific likes and dislikes.

Activities

Activities in the continuing care ward should be so designed as to stimulate the residents and make them feel useful members of society. Interest in the resident's family, past occupation and achievements can do much to raise his spirits and help him to adjust to his new situation. In some units residents' committees have been formed to decide upon the social activities of the unit. These committees usually consist of one or two residents, a therapist, a social worker, some members of the nursing staff and a voluntary worker, and are active in stimulating interest in various activities. The accent should be on living rather than waiting to die.

Knitting, sewing and basketwork are activities commonly associated with the elderly. There is a place for these traditional pursuits of women in the unit and the results can be sold at a coffee morning or bazaar organized on the unit. Some residents enjoy art or specific types of music, such as classical or old-time music hall. Therapy involving music and movement has been developed in some units and this results in extension of the range of the residents' movements and improves their muscle control. An organization known as Sesame has been developing this art amongst sick and handicapped people. Drama has been developed too in some continuing care units. Shape is an arts organization that links professional actors, dancers, musicians, visual artists and writers with people who are physically and mentally disabled, ill, elderly or socially disadvantaged, whether at home or in institutions. The organization believes that the arts fulfil a basic human need, and enable people to express themselves and use their creative capacities to communicate with others.

Educational programmes are being introduced in some units so the elderly can continue to develop their learning skills, which can lead to a feeling of satisfaction and a sense of accomplishment. Many subjects are being pursued, including poetry, drama, current affairs, collage, music and movement, local history, art and craft, and even French conversation. It encourages the elderly to be more mobile and alert and to participate in group activity, helps with improvement in memory and concentration, and gives a sense of identity. The tutors may be supplied from the local education authority, and some branches of the Workers' Education Association or even retired teachers may be recruited to help.

Reminiscence therapy often helps to stimulate the elderly; staff and relatives talking about the past often produces lively conversations of times gone by. One centenarian in my unit visited a local primary school to recount life one hundred years ago and held captive her young audience for some time! Age Concern have produced a series of tape/slide presentations which depict life from the First to the Second World Wars, and when shown to a group of elderly these can stimulate lively discussion.

Equally, reality orientation concentrating on present-day life is important. The elderly should be encouraged to keep abreast of date, day and time. All these should be displayed prominently in the unit. Those who are able should be encouraged to read the newspaper and listen to or watch the news. Television and radio are enjoyed by some, but choice should be given as to which programmes are viewed and neither the radio nor the TV should be left on continuously to disturb all in ward or day areas.

These activities may be enjoyed by a few but should not be

thrust upon the majority who may not wish to participate in all of them. The activities increase the amount of time that the elderly and their carers are involved together and this can only have a good effect on the morale, alertness and general well-being of the elderly residents.

Outings are important and of great benefit to the residents. Access to a coach with a lift is an asset as some residents are too disabled to manoeuvre themselves into a motor car and it is for these that an expedition is so essential. To go out into the countryside, to enjoy the sun and the trees, to visit a theatre or cinema and even to see the sea are activities which we take so much for granted and should not be denied the elderly disabled. It is sometimes possible for visits to be made to a local luncheon club and in some units arrangements are also made for residents to take a holiday. It should be possible for the elderly to do their own shopping and choose their own clothes.

Voluntary workers

Voluntary workers have an important role to play in these units, although they must be carefully selected. The WRVS members who bring round the trolley shop may develop very useful relationships with elderly patients. Some voluntary visitors on a one-to-one basis are often a great support to the elderly person, helping with letter writing, reading and generally conveying news. Schools may send groups of pupils who, if well supervised, can be absorbed and may organize communal games such as bingo or dominoes, and give an hour or two of pleasure to some residents. Volunteers can help run diversional therapy groups and many activities within these units. All visitors from outside are welcome as they all help to provide stimulation and interest.

The occasional party to celebrate a specific event such as Hallowe'en, Christmas or the arrival of strawberries is very popular and a source of amusement. Residents can invite their own guests, help prepare the food and any decorations, and generally become involved in the whole activity. The nurse must remember those elderly who do not appreciate the company of others at all times and enjoy a little solitude. Pets are often an asset, whether dog, cat, budgerigar or fish.

Spiritual needs

The spiritual needs of the elderly must not be forgotten and a good liaison should be kept with the chaplains of various denominations. Religion is, for many people, an important element in their lives from which they derive comfort and inspiration according to the strength of their individual belief.

Clergy should be encouraged to visit the unit and the residents individually and arrangements should be made for residents to attend services in the hospital chapel, or for services to be held in the unit. Sometimes it may be possible for them to attend a local church and to be made to feel a member of the community.

In some areas especially there will be elderly people of other religions who have different customs and diets. There may even be language barriers. There are usually people in the community who will be able to help if there are real difficulties, and families may even contribute to the diet if the hospital is not able to cater for their needs. Every effort should be made to cater for these people in all aspects of daily living and allow them to follow their customs.

The family

Finally, the family should be involved in all activities wherever possible. They should be encouraged to visit frequently and to help with the care of their elderly relative. Sometimes relatives are only too pleased to help with feeding or putting the resident to bed; it gives them a sense of belonging and caring. Invitations to weddings, birthday parties and other family activities should not be withheld from the elderly living in hospital and the nurses should teach the relatives how to manage their own elderly so they can attend these functions and also visit the family home for a meal, a day or even a weekend.

The nurse must not forget the art of communicating with the resident. She must find time to sit and talk, and attempt to understand the feelings of the elderly living within an institution. She must learn to understand their needs, their interests and their problems. It is a demanding job needing perseverance and imagination as there is always room for new ideas when looking after those in the continuing care units.

Younger chronic sick

This unfortunate group of people is still found in continuing care units, although adequate provision is now made for some of them in units of their own; unfortunately these are often far away from their own homes.

In 1970 the Chronically Sick and Disabled Persons Act was passed and this ensured that every local authority was aware of the numbers and needs of the registered disabled living in its area. The local authority should help the disabled and provide facilities to enable them to live at home for as long as possible, if necessary providing special accommodation. When this proves no longer possible or practicable, hospitals must do all they can to ensure that those under 65 are not cared for in wards used for the care of the elderly infirm.

The problems of these younger chronic sick are threefold: physical, psychological and social. Those who find themselves in these units are normally those patients suffering from medical, surgical or neurological conditions, e.g. chronic pulmonary, cardiac or renal conditions, poliomyelitis, muscular dystrophy, multiple sclerosis and severe arthritis.

These patients naturally require special units adapted for their care, with physiotherapy and occupational therapy near at hand. They need to maintain their independence wherever possible and to have every facility for occupation and entertainment available. For them particularly the hospital becomes their home, so privacy should be given them wherever possible, with small rooms available for those who prefer them. Activities need to be therapeutic, and some residents may be able to follow in some way their previous hobbies or professions. Frequent outings and entertainments must be organized.

This type of nursing requires the development of certain skills by the nurse. Great patience is required together with imagination and a sense of humour. The relatives need much support and help, and will be greatly assisted by the help and advice of the social worker. The relatives should be encouraged to visit as often as possible and to partake in the life of the ward and the resident.

Modern trends in continuing care

Care of the elderly handicapped needing continuing nursing care but not requiring the medical and remedial facilities of the district general hospital has posed a problem for some time. The Department of Health and Social Security is currently helping to fund some schemes whereby nursing home care is provided within the National Health Service by smaller units run by nurses. These units will attempt to provide privacy, with residents bringing many of their own possessions including furniture but not beds, freedom of choice in the resident's life-style, and generally a more domestic atmosphere. They will have mainly single rooms with a few double rooms and will accommodate those elderly requiring long-term nursing care. They will not admit those who are terminally ill or need psychiatric treatment, but those who become terminally ill will be able to remain, as will those whose mental states deteriorate, provided they are not too disruptive or require treatment.

This type of care has been successfully given in Scandinavia, especially Denmark, for some years. Here, the elderly requiring long-term nursing care live in state-run Nursing Homes, where each resident has his own room, lavatory, shower and adequate storage space. All the residents are encouraged to furnish their own rooms fully, and the overall impression is of the frail elderly living successfully surrounded by familiar furnishings, and joining together for communal meals and activities.

Further reading

British Geriatrics Society and Royal College of Nursing of the United Kingdom (1975) *Improving Geriatric Care in Hospital.* London: Rcn.

Denham, N. (1983) *Care of the Long Stay Elderly Patient.* London: Croom Helm.

Robb, B. (1967) *Sans Everything.* London: Nelson.

Stewart, M. (1971) *My Brother's Keeper?* London: Health Horizon.

5
Common Diseases of Old Age

When caring for the elderly who are sick, the nurse will come across a variety of diseases, some being more common to old age, while others can be found in people of any age. In order to nurse the patient effectively the nurse must be aware of the cause (where it is known) and the effect the disease can have on the life of the patient, so that the resulting problems can be fully appreciated. When taking the nursing history the nurse will discover for herself many of the problems actually affecting the life of her patient, and a problem-solving approach will be needed when devising the care plan.

DEGENERATIVE DISEASES

Osteoarthritis

Definition
A degenerative arthritis, in which degeneration of the articular cartilage and weight-bearing surfaces of large joints takes place, possibly resulting in shortening of the affected limb. There is no inflammation, and this distinguishes it from rheumatoid arthritis. Also, the disease may affect one or several joints, but not as in rheumatoid arthritis many joints. The common joints affected are the knee, hip and all the weight-bearing joints.

Problems
1 Pain of the affected joint—variable (sometimes slight, sometimes severe) and may radiate, e.g. pain in the hip can radiate down the leg to affect the groin and knee.
2 Restricted movement—the joint becomes stiff and deformed.

Nursing considerations
- Control of pain—adequate and regular analgesia.
- Physiotherapy to improve mobility.
- Weight reductions to halt deterioration.
- Joint replacement if patient is otherwise fit.

Case study—Mrs B. Age 78.

Initial assessment   Mrs B was unable to walk and was wheeled into the ward. Both hips and knees were stiff and painful, and both legs were swollen owing to fluid retention. She only wore slippers as her feet were too swollen for her to wear shoes. She was evidently incontinent as there was a distinctive aroma about her. She was obese.

Pain and discomfort   She had pain in hips and knees, which was worse on movement and in the morning. She found some relief from taking paracetamol or aspirin and a hot-water bottle at night was comforting.

Home circumstances   Mrs B. lived alone in a ground-floor flat. A niece visited weekly. She had a home help daily and lately the community nurse had called daily. She had meals-on-wheels three times a week.

Nursing problems
1 Pain in legs.
2 Difficulty standing.
3 Incontinence of a) urine, b) faeces.
4 Fear she would not get home again.
5 Obesity

Aims of care and action taken
1 *Relief of pain.* Regular analgesia was given and the effect noted.
2 *Ability to stand and move unaided.* A walking-frame was provided and the height of the bed and chair corrected. Mrs B. was encouraged to walk short distance to the lavatory.
3 *Regaining of full continence after 2 weeks.* The nurse responded immediately to requests for toilet. The action of diuretics was explained. Mrs B. was encouraged to walk to the toilet. The toilet seat was checked for correct height.
4 *Reassurance.* The plan to increase mobility and relieve pain was explained.
5 *Reduction of weight by one stone (6 kg).* The nurse liaised with the dietitian, and Mrs B. had the reasons for losing weight explained to her. Good diet was encouraged.

Evaluation after one week
1 Pain improved; analgesia given regularly.
2 Able to stand with walking-frame; lacks confidence.
3 Fully continent as aided to lavatory regularly.
4 Anxious about future.
5 Weight reduction begun.

Evaluation after six weeks
1 Pain minimal; analgesia only required at night.
2 Able to walk with frame—about 50 yards.
3 Fully continent.
4 Going home in 2 weeks; preparations being made, i.e. home visit,
liaison with community nurse.
5 Weight reduction continuing slowly and steadily.

Osteoporosis

Definition
A disease of the bone resulting in reduction of the bone mass,
causing the bone to become more brittle and liable to bend or
fracture. It may be due to low calcium intake or failure to absorb
calcium and it may result from prolonged use of steroids as in
rheumatoid arthritis. It is more common in women than men.

Problems
1 Pain—often in the spine, where the disease most commonly
occurs.
2 Kyphosis—the spine becomes bent, restricting movement.
3 Compression fractures of the vertebral bodies.

Nursing considerations
● Control of pain—adequate analgesia.
● Surgical corset may help the position of the spine.
● Improve mobility and keep patient active for as long as
possible.
● Anabolic steroids may be given, as may calcium supplements.

Osteomalacia

Definition
Softening of the bones due to lack of calcium in the skeleton.
This may be due to vitamin deficiency (lack of vitamin D in the
diet or insufficient exposure to sunlight) or to malabsorption, in

which case steatorrhoea occurs. Also, osteomalacia may occur after a partial gastrectomy.

Problems
1   Pain and weakness affecting the hip and shoulder girdle.
2   Bones become softened and can be painful and tender if pressed.
3   Immobility and difficulty dressing—may be difficult to walk if the pelvic girdle is affected and movement of the arms is restricted if shoulder girdle is affected.

Nursing considerations
- Relief of pain with regular analgesia.
- Vitamin D supplements can be given orally to help improve the condition.
- Physiotherapy and occupational therapy will be helpful once treatment for the disease has commenced.

Paget's disease

Definition
A disease of older people affecting any bone, most commonly the skull, pelvis, clavicle, fibia, femur and vertebrae. The affected bones become larger, thicker and more brittle so are more liable to fracture.

Problems
1   Severe pain.
2   Tendency to fractures.

Treatment
- Relief of pain with analgesia.
- In severe cases the hormone calcitonin may be used.

Cervical spondylosis

Definition
Degeneration or protrusion of the intervertebral discs. It is found in the middle-aged and elderly.

Problems
1   Tingling of arms and hands, occurring especially at night.

2 Weakness and wasting of arms.
3 Pain radiating around the chest wall, neck or back.
4 Difficulty walking and some loss of balance.
5 Vertebrobasilar insufficiency due to degenerative changes in the discs of the neck causing shortening and kinking of the vertebral arteries. Confusion, vertigo and transient loss of consciousness may result.

Nursing considerations
- Use of a plastic collar supporting the neck may be helpful if tolerated.
- Neck traction is not usually applied to the elderly.
- Control of pain with regular analgesia.
- Mobilization with suitable walking-aid. Physiotherapy and occupational therapy to maintain independence in activities of daily living.
- Understanding of the cause of the symptoms and explanation to relatives.

DEFICIENCY DISEASES

Diabetes

Definition
Reduced output of insulin due to decreased pancreatic function, often associated with obesity in old age.

Problems
1 Polyuria (frequency of passing urine even during the night) and polydypsia (thirst).
2 Change of bowel habit and loss of weight.
3 Wounds slow to heal.
4 Peripheral vascular disease with resulting gangrene.
5 Diabetic neuropathy.
6 Ocular disorders including disorders of the retina and formation of cataracts.

Nursing considerations
- Urine should be tested regularly to note control of diabetes and give suitable fluids when required. Medical treatment of diabetes by insulin initially and then oral hypoglycaemics should be carefully monitored by the nurse and urine or blood

may be tested 4-hourly. A chart should be kept of the results. The oral hypoglycaemics generally used are chlorpropamide, metformin or glibenclamide.

- A suitable diet should be prescribed and adhered to. This may be initiated by the dietitian and the nurse must ensure that the patient fully understands the necessity for this and what it entails. The relatives too should be involved and encourage the patient to stick to his diet. Many elderly people will only require control of their diabetes by diet alone, especially those who are obese and will find such a diet hard to follow!

- Once a diet and treatment have been commenced the other problems should slowly improve. Care should be taken of any wounds but they should heal slowly when the blood sugar is under control.

- Care should be taken of all extremities. Toe-nails should be cut by the chiropodist as any injury to the foot may have long-lasting effects. After washing, the feet should always be dried very carefully and care should be taken of heels and ankles.

- Many long-term diabetic patients have poor sight and help should be given to adapt to this condition.

Case study—Mrs J. Age 84.

Initial assessment   Mrs J. was a well-built lady but had obviously lost some weight recently as her clothes all hung loosely. She was able to walk with a stick, but had a painful ulcer on her leg which was failing to heal.

Reason patient gave for admission   She was found to have sugar in her urine by the community nurse, who had done a routine urine test when visiting to dress her leg ulcer. As she was losing weight and passing large amounts of urine, it was felt that the diabetes would be easier to stabilize in hospital.

Pain and discomfort   The patient complained of continual thirst, of having to pass urine frequently and of having to get up at night to do so too. She had noticed that she had been losing weight and lately her stools were more frequent and less formed. Her sight had deteriorated over the past 2 years.

Home circumstances   Mrs J. lived alone. Her son, who lived nearby, visited twice weekly and her neighbours were friendly. She had meals-on-wheels twice weekly and a home help once a week. The community nurse had been visiting three times weekly to dress her leg ulcer.

Nursing problems
1 Thirst and polyuria.
2 Ulcer which was failing to heal.
3 Poor sight.

Aims of care and action taken
1 *Relief of thirst and polyuria.* The nurse liaised with the doctor in the treatment of the patient's diabetes. Mrs J. was given metformin 500 mg before breakfast and before supper. Her urine was tested 4-hourly by the nurse and recorded on her chart. The blood sugar was recorded daily by the doctor and control was quickly attained.
2 *Dietary control.* Mrs J. was seen by the dietitian and the importance of carbohydrates was explained to her. As Mrs J. was mentally very alert she was able to grasp this. She was provided with some literature to guide her. Her son was also seen by the dietitian.
3 *Healing of ulcer.* The wound was cleaned daily with Eusol and a dry dressing applied. Once the diabetes was controlled, improvement was noted.
4 *Improvement of eyesight.* Mrs J. was seen by the Consultant Ophthalmologist, who confirmed early cataracts. She was introduced to large-print books, and later on a home visit the lighting was examined and improved in places. All loose mats were removed and she was given a large number dial for her telephone.

Evaluation after 1 week
1 No longer thirsty and passing less urine. Urine tests were either negative or 0.25%.
2 Mrs J. had grasped the importance of her diet and was following it closely.
3 The ulcer had started to heal.
4 Mrs J. was enjoying reading again.

Evaluation after 6 weeks
1 Mrs J. was at home again coping well. Her urine was tested daily by herself and was nearly always negative.
2 She enjoyed her diet and was able to follow it closely.
3 Her leg ulcer had healed.

Hypothyroidism or myxoedema

Definition
Reduction in output of thyroxine by the thyroid gland, which is in turn controlled by the pituitary gland.

Problems
1 Sensitivity to cold—the patient often has a considerably lowered body temperature.
2 Lethargy leading to coma.
3 Rough, dry skin.
4 Confusion.
5 Anaemia.
6 Weight gain.
7 Tendency to falls.
8 Cramp at night.
9 Deep hoarse voice and slow speech.

Medical treatment
Thyroid function test will confirm diagnosis. Thyroxine will be administered to ensure the correct level of the hormone in the body. It can lead to cardiac failure and care should be taken to avoid this.

Nursing considerations
Most of the problems will resolve themselves with the administration of thyroxine. Any signs of heart failure should be reported.

Anaemia

Definition
A low haemoglobin level, i.e. 12 g/dl of blood or less. This is most common amongst the elderly and there are several causes. The elderly person will appear pale and the mucous membranes are also very pale.

Iron deficiency or microcytic anaemia

Problems
These are now always easy to define if the anaemia is of slow onset:
1 Tiredness, breathlessness on exertion.
2 Headaches, lack of concentration.
3 Palpitations, swollen ankles.
4 Confusion.
5 If the haemoglobin has been low for some time, then

problems include brittle nails, smooth tongue and cracking at the corners of the mouth.

Medical treatment
The cause of the anaemia should be ascertained and subsequent treatment should involve either iron supplements or if necessary a blood transfusion. The most common causes of iron deficiency anaemia are chronic blood loss from hiatus hernia, carcinoma of the stomach or colon, diverticulitis, haemorrhoids, dietary insufficiency, and drugs, e.g. aspirin and other anti-inflammatory agents.

Nursing considerations
- Help establish the cause, i.e. collect stools for occult blood and help with other tests.
- Help with replacement therapy, i.e. administration of iron or blood. Iron may be given intravenously, but this is not often done. Jectofer (iron sorbitol) and Imferon (iron dextran) may be given intramuscularly; Jectofer is more quickly absorbed, but less Imferon is excreted in the urine. Also, there are many preparations of iron that can be given orally. Some are released slowly, and some combined with ascorbic acid for more efficient absorption. Some can cause gastric upsets. The patients should be warned that their stools will be black.
- Improve the diet—the patient should understand the value of foods containing iron being added to the diet (e.g. red meat, liver, egg yolk, spinach), and they should be encouraged to enjoy them.

Vitamin B_{12} and folic acid deficiency, or macrocytic anaemia

Macrocytic anaemia is the most common anaemia seen in the elderly. Vitamin B_{12} deficiency is due to achlorhydria preventing the absorption of vitamin B_{12}. Folic acid deficiency is due to lack of folic acid in the diet.

Problems
The onset is slow and problems are not apparent until the anaemia is severe:
1 Lemon tinge to the skin.
2 Sore tongue.

3   Numbness and tingling of hands and feet.
4   Swelling of ankles and breathlessness due to heart failure.

Nursing considerations
● Replacement therapy. In the case of vitamin B12 deficiency,
  the vitamin is administered by injection, daily initially, then
  weekly, monthly and finally 3-monthly. Folic acid may be
  given in oral form. It may also be found in liver and green
  vegetables.

INFLAMMATORY DISEASES

Rheumatoid arthritis

Definition
A disease usually affecting symmetrical joints causing swelling
and joint effusions. The joint surfaces become infiltrated, the
cartilage breaks up and joint space is lost.

Problems
1   Pain, stiffness of affected joints.
2   Local inflammation and swelling of affected joints.
3   Limitation of movement.
4   General malaise and depression.
5   Loss of weight.
6   Tiredness

Nursing considerations
● Relief of pain. Effective analgesia should be given and at
  regular intervals so that the patient can move without undue
  discomfort. Paracetamol is preferable to aspirin, which
  causes gastrointestinal haemorrhage due to gastric irritation
  and occasional hypersensitivity. Steroids may occasionally be
  used but are not often justifiable for long-term use for the
  elderly patient. Short courses of high dosage may be beneficial while the disease is active.
● Increase in movement so that the patient can lead as active a
  life as possible without too much discomfort. A balance has to
  be found between rest and movement. Rest in bed may be
  necessary at first. The nurse and the physiotherapist must
  ensure that there is good position of all the joints. Padded
  splints or light plastic casts may be used.

- Passive movements may be commenced as soon as possible and eventually the patient will graduate to activities of daily living encouraged by the nurse, physiotherapist and occupational therapist. Patients who have severe deformities of the joints after years of suffering from rheumatoid arthritis are often seen in the geriatric unit. These patients generally have a low pain threshold. Some help may be given by gentle exercises, possibly preceded by wax baths. Little improvement will be expected in mobility but eventually the patient may be helped by specially designed aids.

- The general health of the patient can be improved by encouraging a good diet with plenty of rest. Many old people living alone tend to make do with bread and butter and cups of tea. The patient may need help with cutting up solid food if the hands are deformed and painful. The doctor will ensure that anaemia and possible vitamin and mineral deficiencies are corrected with the appropriate supplements. Emphasis should be placed upon red meats, milk, eggs and fresh fruit. It is often necessary in hospital to add iron, ascorbic acid, folic acid, multivitamins and calcium to the medication.

Temporal arteritis

Definition
A disease affecting medium-sized arteries, often branches of the external caratoid artery. It occurs more commonly as people get older.

Problems
1 The temporal artery becomes tender, hot and thickened in the acute stage, and as a result the patient complains of headache.
2 The patient feels generally unwell, weak and tired.
3 The retinal artery may be affected and this will cause impaired or total loss of vision.

Nursing considerations
- As the ESR is raised, steroids should be commenced, 40–60 mg daily initially, reduced fairly quickly but maintained over the following year.
- Where vision is affected, much reassurance and help will be required of the nurse.

Polymyalgia rheumatica

Definition
A disease affecting the muscles of the limb girdles.

Problems
1 Pain and weakness of the shoulder and pelvic girdle.
2 General weakness and malaise.
3 Pyrexia and raised ESR.

Treatment
● Treatment by steroids is again necessary and results are often very good with quite dramatic improvement.

HEART DISEASE

Congestive heart failure

Definition
A common disability of old age for which there are many causes, the most common being ischaemic heart disease, but including anaemia and occasionally thyrotoxicosis or myxoedema. It may be precipitated by disease of the lungs such as chronic bronchitis.

Problems
1 Dyspnoea and orthopnoea.
2 Cough is nearly always present.
3 Patient complains of weakness and lassitude.
4 Confusion and agitation.
5 Insomnia and nocturnal restlessness due to an inadequate supply of oxygen to the brain.
6 Oedema of feet and ankles.
7 Immobility.
8 Lack of appetite.

Nursing considerations
● The problems with breathing are often improved by good positioning of the patient. If he is nursed upright and the pillows are well placed this may help to relieve the situation. Administration of digoxin and a diuretic by the doctor will also help to improve breathing problems.

- Cough can be relieved by a soothing linctus. Diuretics too may help to relieve the cough.
- Weakness and lassitude improve as the general condition of the patient improves.
- Confusion and agitation may be relieved if the patient is nursed in familiar surroundings with possessions and people around that he can recognize.
- Insomnia can be improved if the patient is nursed upright in bed. Sedation should be avoided if possible but a warm drink may be given. Keeping a night-light by the patient may also help to relieve agitation and confusion. Sometimes these patients prefer to sleep in a chair.
- Oedema of feet and ankles will be improved with diuretics. The patient should be encouraged to sit with his feet up when possible and the foot of the bed should be elevated at night.
- The patient should be encouraged to take a little exercise, to sit out in a chair and if possible walk to the lavatory.
  Small appetizing meals, attractively presented should be offered and nutritious drinks supplied. Salt restriction is necessary for all patients with heart failure and in severe cases salt should not be added to the cooking. Unfortunately, most patients with congestive heart failure lack an appetite and this restriction of salt does not help the palatability of food.
- Digitalis is nearly always given in these cases as it slows and strengthens the heart beat, and controls atrial fibrillation which may be present. Old people are often very sensitive to this drug, and the nurse should record the pulse before giving the dosage. The doctor must be informed if it is abnormally slow or irregular. The normal dose of digoxin is 0.25 mg once or twice daily; usually digoxin PG (paediatric/geriatric) will be given 0.0625 mg twice daily as old people tend to be so sensitive. Digoxin may also cause nausea and vomiting. Sensitivity to digoxin is frequently aggravated by hypokalaemia caused by the use of diuretics. Nevertheless, diuretics may be needed and the type used may depend upon the patient's ability to control the act of micturition. Frusemide 40–80 mg orally or 40 mg by intramuscular injection gives a rapid result, its action only lasting four hours. Moduretic, however, has a slower action and may be more beneficial to those with a tendency to incontinence. It may be necessary to change the diuretic from time to time, as it may cease to be effective. A potassium supplement will be given with some diuretics as potassium is lost in the urine.

Cerebrovascular disease

There are reported to be 100 000–120 000 new cases of cerebrovascular accident every year, and 75% of these occur in the over-65 age group. There is thought to be a 50% survival rate after the first 'stroke'.

There are three main types of cerebrovascular disease:
1 cerebral thrombosis
2 cerebral haemorrhage
3 cerebral embolism.

Cerebral thrombosis

This may be due to a sudden fall in blood pressure or some blood disorder. The thrombosis may take place at rest or when sleeping, often extending over a few hours ot days. The onset is gradual with drowsiness followed by loss of consciousness or a fit.

Cerebral haemorrhage

This may be caused by uncontrolled, possibly unsuspected, hypertension, or by a bleeding disorder. The patient is often in a coma on arrival at hospital, the onset being very sudden, frequently with loss of consciousness, and death may follow rapidly.

Cerebral embolism

This occurs commonly in the patient with atrial fibrillation or bacterial endocarditis. As in cerebral haemorrhage the onset is sudden and the degree of disability is obvious immediately.

Problems
These vary according to the severity of the stroke. Some of the difficulties encountered are as follows:
1 Loss of use of a limb or limbs.
2 Loss of speech or difficulty with speech. Aphasia is total absence of speech, and dysarthria is imperfect articulation due to a mechanical fault of some kind.
3 Apraxia (failure to recognize common articles and their use).
4 Visual defects such as hemianopia (loss of part of the visual field).

5   Difficulty swallowing.
6   Emotional disturbances—signs of aggression and depression, difficulty in communication and lack of motivation.

Nursing considerations
- Treatment of the affected limb or limbs—ensure correct support in bed so that no deformity takes place (see Fig. 12). Once the patient is up, he should again be correctly supported and physiotherapy will commence quite quickly. The nurse must be aware of the active and passive movements given as she must carry these out over the 24 hour period. The occupational therapist will also teach the patient how to cope with the affected side and how to dress, feed and so on independently where possible. Sometimes the patient will reject the affected side and fail to acknowledge that it is there.

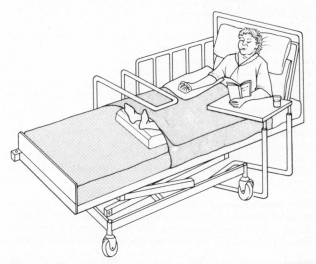

Figure 12. Correct position of hemiplegic patient in bed.

- Where there are speech problems, the speech therapist will be asked to see the patient and will plan a programme to help with his individual needs. The nurse must be aware of this and help to carry out the programme over the 24 hours. The relatives too should be involved with all the remedial therapists.

- Visual defects may improve with exercise. Articles should be placed within the patient's visual field but the patient should be encouraged to practise extending his field with exercises.
- Swallowing difficulties should be assessed and food should be prepared that is suitable for the individual patient's needs. If necessary an emulsified or liquid diet can be given.
- Much support and understanding needs to be given to the patient during this period. The relatives too will need much help. Activities need to be planned by the nurse to keep the patient motivated and alert. In many cases the progress is slow and improvement is gradual, and morale must be high for the patient to continue to strive to maintain his improvement.

Case study—Mrs D. Age 68.

Initial assessment   Mrs D. was admitted to the geriatric unit from home having had a cerebrovascular accident three weeks previously, leaving her with a left hemiplegia. She looked rather depressed, her left arm hung loosely at her side, and she had an obvious left-sided flaccid weakness and some difficulty with speech not aided by ill-fitting dentures. When she transferred into an armchair it was noted that she had weakness of her left leg also.

Reason patient gave for admission   Since her stroke, she had had considerable difficulty managing at home. Her daughter had come in frequently but was exhausted and Mrs D. felt she was making no progress. She felt she might well not be able to live alone again and this depressed her greatly.

Pain and discomfort   Mrs D. was considerably limited by her left-sided weakness and found it difficult to cope with. Her ill-fitting dentures were an embarrassment. She was constipated, not having opened her bowels for two weeks, and this left her with a poor appetite.

Home circumstances   Mrs D. lived alone. When she was fit she was independent, although she saw her daughter and young family regularly. She lived in a convenient ground-floor flat. She was a sociable lady—she attended the local old people's club and had helped to run it for some time.

Nursing problems
1   Immobility due to weakness.

2   Constipation.
3   Ill-fitting dentures plus dysarthria.
4   Depression.

Aims of care and action taken
1   *Improvement of mobility with exercise.* She was referred to the physiotherapist and occupational therapist and rehabilitation was continued 24 hours a day.
2   *Relief of constipation.* Fluids and a good diet were encouraged. Bran was added to the diet.
3   *Replacement of dentures.* An appointment was made with a dentist. She was also referred to a speech therapist for exercises to help in overcoming the dysarthria.
4   *Improvement in morale.* The aims of care and her progress were explained to her.

Evaluation after one week
1   Mrs D. was able to transfer from bed to chair and chair to lavatory unaided. She had started walking with the aid of the physiotherapist and her tripod. She had regained much confidence.
2   Her bowels were working normally aided by ample fluids and a good diet with added bran.
3   A dental appointment had been made for the next week. She had seen a speech therapist.
4   Morale was high as she could see she was making progress.

Evaluation after six weeks
1   Mrs D. was walking and dressing unaided.
2   Her bowels were normal.
3   Her teeth had been adjusted. With exercise her speech had much improved.
4   Morale was very high. She was going home next week, to attend the day hospital twice weekly initially. She was to have a home help once weekly and meals-on-wheels when she was not in the day hospital, except for weekends when her daughter would help. She was determined to do her own cooking and housework as soon as possible.

CHEST DISEASES

Acute or chronic bronchitis

Definitions
Chronic bronchitis is brought about by the degeneration of lung tissue, which causes an increase in the amount of mucoid bronchial secretions, resulting in daily expectoration. Acute

bronchitis occurs when there is infective exacerbation of this condition. The incidence of the disease is high in the United Kingdom, particularly in northern industrial areas where the climate is cold and damp. It is also more commonly seen in the obese patient and it is aggravated by smoking.

Problems
1 Breathlessness on exertion.
2 Persistent cough.
3 Lethargy and general malaise.
4 Obesity.

Nursing considerations
- Bronchial dilators may be used, e.g. salbutamol or Choledyl (choline theophyllinate). Make sure the patient sleeps in a fairly upright position with adequate pillows.
- Cough linctus may be prescribed and a warm drink at night may help.

Pneumonia

Definition
Inflammation of the lung. It is often difficult to diagnose as signs other than the reactive development in the lung present themselves. It is the most common cause of death in the elderly, especially following bronchitis, cerebrovascular accident, congestive cardiac failure and fractured femur.

Problems
1 Breathlessness and tachycardia.
2 Restlessness and confusion.
3 Lack of appetite and dehydration.

Nursing considerations
- Nurse upright in bed or chair. Administer antibiotic if prescribed—often a broad spectrum antibiotic such as Vibramycin (doxycycline) is used. Keep warm.
- Try to keep as well orientated as possible with familiar objects around.
- Encourage nourishing fluids and light meals. Complan, Build-Up and fresh fruit juice should be used.

HYPOTHERMIA

Definition
Body temperature falls below 35°C (normal body temperature is 37°C).

    34°–35°C—mild hypothermia
    30°–34°C—moderate hypothermia
        30°C—severe hypothermia.

Primary cause is dysfunction of the body's temperature-regulating system. Secondary causes are underlying disease, e.g. endocrine disorders, immobility, poor circulation, neurological disease, and excessive sedation and use of anti-depressants. Accidental hypothermia occurs when there is prolonged exposure to extreme cold due to cold weather, accidents at home, or financial problems leading to inadequate heating, loneliness and apathy.

Problems
1 Cold—the patient feels cold, is sluggish in movement, and may be shivering.
2 Slow pulse, hypotension and a slow circulation.
3 Very shallow respiration—pneumonia may develop.

Nursing considerations
- Warm the patient very slowly, and nurse in a warm room with adequate blankets. Do not overheat as this can cause too rapid warming, in which case the blood pressure may fall and the circulation fail, possibly leading to pneumonia and death. It may be necessary to use a foil blanket, which provides good insulation and prevents heat escaping.
- Give nourishing warm drinks and maintain fluid intake.
- Course of steroids may be given in severe cases. Recovery should be evident in 12 hours.
- Take note of the cause of hypothermia. Those who have become cold due to financial problems may need help with benefits. Three quarters of those receiving supplementary benefit are eligible for help with heating costs. It is estimated that about one million people are at risk from hypothermia every winter (*Nursing Times*, 1983).

PARKINSONISM

Definition
Structural or biochemical alterations within the basal ganglia of the brain affecting the metabolism of dopamine. It affects about 1% of the population over the age of 60 in some form or other. It may be due to arteriosclerosis or may be drug induced, usually by the phenothiazine group of drugs.

Problems
1   Akinesia—an abnormal absence or reduction of muscular movement caused by paralysis of the motor nerves resulting in difficulty in initiating voluntary movement.
2   Tremor. This occurs unpreceded by any other symptom. It affects resting muscles and may initially affect only one upper limb. It is absent during sleep and is greatly exacerbated by anxiety. It may also be halted by voluntary movement of the affected limb.
3   Rigidity often appears in the early stages of the disease in the form of severe cramp, and then develops into a resistance to passive movement, either constant ('lead pipe') or intermittent ('cog wheel').
4   Dysphagia—difficulty in swallowing associated with general flexion in posture including neck and shoulders.
5   Immobility. The patient has a characteristic gait caused by a combination of rigidity, akinesia and associated difficulty in balance. The patient moves by short steps, accelerating as if trying to keep up with his centre of gravity, with the arms kept to the sides instead of swinging.

Nursing considerations
● Much depends on the patient's response to chemotherapy. The introduction of levodopa into the treatment of parkinsonism has made management far easier as it is most effective in controlling tremor, rigidity and akinesia. It has to be given in large doses as it is destroyed in the gut and may cause nausea and vomiting. This may be alleviated if given with food. Other side-effects include hypotension, depression, abnormal voluntary movements and paranoia. It may be combined with other drugs such as orphenadrine.
● Physiotherapy and occupational therapy play a large part in

treating these patients. The nurse must co-operate with the therapists so that treatment can continue 24 hours a day.

- Much encouragement and ingenuity needs to be used by the nursing staff to overcome many of the difficulties encountered by these patients. Many of them are mentally very alert and are fully aware of their difficulties.

- Relatives need much support and help. When patients are at home they may well require constant attention and need much patience and understanding. In some areas support groups have been formed by the Parkinson Disease Society. This society offers help and support for both the sufferer and his relatives.

Case study—Mr N. Age 84

Initial assessment   Mr N. appeared depressed, lacking facial expression and motivation. He had a tremor affecting his left arm and some rigidity of all limbs. He walked with a shuffling gait and had difficulty initiating the process. He was obviously incontinent at times as his clothes were soiled and there was a poor odour. He had obviously lost weight as his clothes were loose!

Reason patient gave for admission   He didn't know why he had been admitted, except he felt the home no longer wanted him. He complained of nothing except feeling depressed and wishing to die.

Home circumstances   He lived in a county council old people's home, having been there for 5 years. Initially he had been quite active, even pottering in the garden, but recently had become rather immobile and morose. He had become incontinent as he could not walk to the lavatory and refused to use a urinal. He had been a schoolmaster at the local secondary school and used to enjoy reading and even doing a little writing, but not in the past year.

Nursing problems
1 Immobility due to condition.
2 Incontinence due to immobility.
3 Apathy with regard to food and loss of weight.
4 Failure to read and take interest in life.

Aims of care and action taken
1 *Encouragement of mobility.* One capsule of Madopar 62.5 was given three times a day and one tablet of Sinemet-110 was added three times a day after 10 days. Physiotherapy and occupational therapy were

commenced at once. The nurse was able to help him out of his chair and to walk with a frame.

2 *Maintenance of continence.* After successful encouragement, he was able to walk to the lavatory and was not incontinent. The fly buttons on his trousers were replaced with Velcro so he could manage the whole affair himself. Being a confirmed bachelor he hated any interference of this kind.

3 *Improvement of appetite and gain in weight.* He was provided with adaptations to cutlery and his plate so he could eat unaided. He enjoyed sherry before meals and his appetite improved. He hated being fed or making a mess but with these aids he could eat cleanly and independently.

4 *Improvement in morale and stimulation of interest.* His morale slowly improved and he took to reading the daily paper and borrowed books from the library. The son of a neighbouring patient was one of his ex-pupils and took great interest in his progress.

Evaluation after six weeks

1 Mr N. returned to the home after 3 weeks and continued to attend the day hospital for 6 weeks on a weekly basis to monitor progress.

2 He could walk well with a frame and was quite independent in all activities of daily living. The tremor remained a problem when he was agitated.

3 He had gained weight and enjoyed his food.

4 He was once again taking an interest in life, reading and pottering in the garden.

URINARY TRACT INFECTION

Definition

Infection affecting any part of the urinary tract, including the kidneys. This is common in men and women over the age of 65, with a higher incidence in old people's homes and geriatric units. As the elderly become more immobile the incidence of urinary tract infections appears to rise. This may be due to (a) constipation and faecal incontinence causing soiling of the perineum and introduction of infection into the urethra, (b) constipation leading to incomplete emptying of the bladder, or (c) abnormalities of the bladder, e.g. enlarged prostate gland in male patients.

Problems

1 Frequency, urgency and dysuria.

2   Dehydration because patient is reluctant to drink.
3   Poor hygiene.

Nursing considerations
- Encourage frequent visits to the lavatory, making patient feel relaxed and able to pass urine whenever he needs.
- Encourage frequent nourishing drinks and explain the importance of this.
- Encourage good hygiene and frequent washing of the perineum where the patient is incontinent.

Frequent urinary tract infections may eventually lead to uraemia. The patient becomes increasingly drowsy, the skin dry and tongue furred. In many cases it may be necessary to give intravenous fluids initially to restore hydration and the electrolyte balance.

NEOPLASTIC DISEASE

Neoplastic disease is relatively common in the elderly, especially carcinoma of the breast, stomach, colon, prostate gland, skin, lungs and bones. Age is not generally a contra-indication to surgery, provided the patient has no other serious disease. The surgeon will operate on the elderly patient in order to relieve distressing symptoms and enable the patient to lead as active a life as possible and not to be a burden on the relatives. Much depends on the patient's physical ability and his outlook and attitude to life, and also that of the relatives. Radiotherapy and chemotherapy may play a part in treatment, although many neoplasms in the elderly are not radiosensitive. Courses of chemotherapeutic treatment are long, often with unpleasant side-effects, and again are not suitable in this age group, except in selected cases.

MULTIPLE PATHOLOGY

It is rare for a patient to be admitted to the geriatric unit with only one disease or disorder. Those elderly who live at home have an average of three disorders, and those who come into hospital may have four or five disorders. Each disease is not lethal by itself but throws a strain on other systems, the accumulative effect causing disability. Acute illness superimposed upon a chronic disability leads to breakdown and crisis. Frequently the patient admitted with severe osteoarthrosis of the hips for a period of rehabilitation may have anaemia due to poor absorption of iron and vitamin B12 and also osteoporosis of the spine. In addition to this he may have haemorrhoids causing considerable discomfort, poor sight such as presbyopia (natural changes that take place in the eyes with advancing age affecting the power of accommodation and resulting in poor sight, which can be improved with new glasses), and presbycussis, i.e. excessive wax in the ear resulting in poor hearing. Hence it can be seen that it is necessary for every patient to have a thorough nursing assessment and a thorough clinical examination on admission. It is important that all aspects of the patient's care, i.e. nursing, medical and social, are covered while the patient is in hospital.

FALLS

Falls are common for the elderly and are often a cause of admission to hospital, and delay the patient's progress when in hospital through injury or loss of confidence. Many can be prevented, although falls are to be expected when advocating and encouraging independence. Patients especially prone to falls are taught how to fall, and how to stand up again unaided if necessary. The most common result is fracture of the upper end of the femur. There are three common causes of falls:

Loss of consciousness
This group includes patients with transient cerebral ischaemic attacks or those who have small infarcts due to cerebral emboli, and also those with a vertigo or syncope which may be due to a tranquillizer or the sudden onset of anaemia, and those with postural hypotension. Into this group also come those patients with epilepsy, which often presents in the hemiplegic patient or patient with multiple 'small strokes'.

Loss of balance
This affects those patients with parkinsonism, in which there is a failure of muscle co-ordination usually due to diseases of the cerebellum including vertebrobasilar artery insufficiency.

Included in this group are those patients suffering from the effect of certain drugs or overdosage of drugs which should be noted by the nurse. Those to be especially observed are certain tranquillizers, hypertensive drugs, levodopa and many types of night sedation which may cause the patient to become confused and lose balance when rising at night. Also included in this group are those patients who suffer from cough syncope or micturition syncope. This is caused by transitory cerebral anaemia due to the effect of straining and the latter is particularly common in elderly men with enlarged prostate, the syncope generally occurring at night when the patient gets up to go to the commode or lavatory. Loss of balance may also occur as a result of poor footcare. Long horny toe-nails, untreated corns and bunions result in the patient wearing unsuitable footwear which gives little support.

Tripping

This group is the most preventable and the nurse can do much to overcome and eradicate these falls. The fall may be due to poor eyesight and therefore there should be good illumination with no deep shadows, especially on stairs and steps. Loose door mats and unnecessary rugs should be removed. Footwear should be examined, and the patient encouraged to wear leather or rope-soled shoes which give good support. Slippers may be abandoned. Night sedation should be reduced, with no barbiturates; chloral or chloral derivatives only should be given. For every patient optimum fitness and mobility should be achieved so that falls are reduced to a minimum.

Fractured femur

Patients are frequently seen following treatment of a fractured femur in the orthopaedic ward, when they progress to the geriatric unit for rehabilitation. It must be remembered that the fracture is often the cause and not the result of the fall. A fracture may occur if the patient turns suddenly, no matter how carefully, when the bones are osteoporotic.

There are two main types of fracture:
a   *Subcapital*, which is unsatisfactory to treat and is followed by a 40% morbidity. It is treated by removal of the femoral head and insertion of a prosthesis. Early mobilization is essential.

b   *Intratrochanteric* which is far more satisfactory to treat with better results being achieved. It is treated with a pin and plate repair and early mobilization is much easier to achieve.

Problems
1   Effects of local injury.
2   Effects of the elderly being immobilized and undergoing general anaesthesia.
3   Complications which arise may include pneumonia, development of pressure sores, urinary tract infection, uraemia, pulmonary embolism and deep vein thrombosis.
4   In the case of insertion of a prosthesis, eventually the prosthesis may become dislocated or burrow into the pelvis.

Nursing considerations
● The nurse must observe all the rules applied to the immobile elderly and encourage mobilization as soon as possible.

Because of the problems of a general anaesthetic in the elderly, some successful experiments have been undertaken by immediate pinning under local anaesthetic, with the patient up and walking straight away, and being discharged from hospital after 48 hours. It must be remembered that, in encouraging a patient's mobilization and independence, a fractured femur is a possible hazard of progress in this direction. However, this is far outweighed by the numerous ill effects following prolonged bed rest and over protectiveness. The increasing problem of the fractured femur in the elderly female has prompted the development of combined geriatric/orthopaedic wards.

POLYPHARMACY

The danger of improper use of drugs by the elderly is far greater at home where there may be no supervision. Although overdoses of drugs may be taken, it is just as likely that medication may be omitted altogether. Night sedation may be a danger as the dose may be repeated if the patient wakes in the night. The old should have simplified drug schedules with clearly labelled containers. Many practise self-medication with favourite remedies often unknown to their medical advisers.

The nurse can do much to help the doctor regulate the dosage and note any side-effects such as vomiting, nausea, loss of balance, falls, dizziness, excessive drowsiness and confusion. Drugs supplied to the elderly should be reduced to an absolute minimum.

References

Oliver, C. (1983) Old and cold. *Nursing Times* (Oct.).
Saddington, M. (1983) Winter of discontent. *Nursing Times* (Oct.).

Further reading

Ferguson Anderson, Sir W., Caird, F.I., Kennedy, R.D. & Schwartz, D. (1982) *Gerontology and Geriatric Nursing*. London: Hodder and Stoughton.
Hall, M.R.P., Maclennan, W.J. & Lye, M.D.W. (1978) *Medical Care of the Elderly*. Oxford: HM+M.
Irvine, R.E. (1984) The Hastings approach—the patient with femoral neck fracture. *Brit. J. Geriat. Nurs.* Vol. 3 (No. 3), p. 12.
Mitchell, R.G. (1984) Falls in the elderly. *Nursing Times* (Jan.).
Wilcock, G.K. & Middleton, A.M. (1980) *Geriatrics*. London: Grant McIntyre.

6
Maintenance of Continence

The promotion of continence is an important part of the nurse's role whilst caring for elderly patients. There are many different aspects to this role and these will be discussed in the following chapter. It has been shown (Wells, 1980) that on those wards where the most time was spent promoting continence, the incidence of incontinence was lowest, but interestingly enough on those wards where incontinence was in fact highest (i.e. continuing care wards), the time spent on promoting continence was least! More time was spent on the palliative work of changing sheets and pads. Thus we may conclude that the more effort and enthusiasm put into the job by the nursing staff, the more rewarding are the results.

Incontinence is a failure to control the evacuation of the bladder or bowel, and is generally associated with elderly patients, although it can affect any age group and causes great distress to the sufferers. There are known to be over three million people incontinent in this country at any one time and 25% of people over the age of 70 are incontinent. Twelve per cent of the elderly living at home are fairly frequently incontinent, 50% of those living in hospital and 48% of those living in private nursing homes (Wade *et al.*, 1983), so it can be seen that the problem produces a challenge to those caring for these people. It costs £5 000 000 a year on pads alone, so it is not only a drain on health resources but also causes much misery to all those suffering from the consequences.

The bladder is a highly sensitive organ and often a person's emotional state can be determined by his bladder function. Hence it is very important that the nurse's attitude is geared towards creating the right atmosphere in which to treat the patient. If the nurse is able to create a warm, relaxed atmosphere where patients and relatives can feel at ease, all patients will respond well and be greatly helped. Good communication between nurse and patient is of vital importance also. The individualized approach to care as advocated in the nursing process is an essential part of caring for the elderly, especially those who are incontinent. The information gained while taking the nursing history will include problems of bladder and bowel function, although it may take some time to extract some of the details from patients, who are often reluctant to discuss these problems or who refuse to admit their existence.

When treating the elderly, privacy and dignity should be preserved at all times. It is important that lavatories should be used wherever possible and that these should be readily accessible, warm and clean, and in well designed units these are within 10 m (40 feet) of patient areas. Rails should be there to help the disabled and access should be easy. If the patient is unable to reach the lavatory, a commode should be used in privacy and especially at night. Bedpans should only be used as a very last resort, preferably not at all. Rigid commode rounds should not be strictly adhered to and the patient should be encouraged to visit the lavatory whenever he feels the necessity.

Keeping the patients active and motivated will help to improve the situation and the importance of wearing their own clothes must be stressed here, as this will raise the morale of the ward and lower the incidence of incontinence. In many units a personalized clothing system with laundry on site is the norm so that all patients wear their own clothes, including underwear. Patients should never be left to sit in an open-backed night-gown on an incontinence pad. Pants should be worn at all times during the day unless the patient specifically requests that these are omitted for some personal reason.

Incontinence in the home may be the final factor in producing a crisis which forces the relatives to find accommodation for their elderly person elsewhere. The elderly may seek to disguise their inability to control bladder or bowel function and not infrequently may hide their soiled clothing, causing considerable distress to themselves and to the relatives with whom they are living. Ignorance of the help that can be obtained for incontinent patients and their families is still very prevalent among the general public despite the fact that more effort is put into publicizing incontinence aids in doctors' surgeries and chemist shops. Laundry services are available in many local authorities. There are a variety of pants and pads obtainable for those with only occasional incontinence and many different coverings for the bed. The Easinurse Mattress on a specially adapted bed has its uses for the mentally alert but immobile patient, as it has a hole in the middle for a receiver, and provided the patient is positioned correctly, may stay dry for some time. For the immobile man it is often adequate to leave in position a urinal which may be fitted with a non-spill valve, but for those who are up and ambulant, there are various types of condom available which, attached to rubber tubing, drain into a bag attached to the leg. Clothing is important, as previously stressed, and there are various specialities available too—short vests, washable Terylene trousers, trousers with Velcro openings, dresses with a split down the back and an overlapping skirt. Nowadays, with efficient pads and pants available, it is possible for the elderly to wear their own clothes and for them not to become soiled.

Incontinence must be viewed objectively as a disability which can be investigated, treated and in most cases alleviated in one way or another.

The nurse plays the most important part in the promotion of continence, and in order that she can carry out her work effectively, she must understand some of its causes.

Normal micturition

Normal micturition occurs when nervous impulses from the stretched muscle wall of the bladder travel to the sacral cord, and impulses travel via the parasympathetic nervous system to the bladder causing the muscle to contract and the sphincter to relax. In the healthy person this is also governed by impulses from the brain transmitted via the sympathetic nervous system so that the bladder is emptied at a convenient time in the right place. The normal healthy person does not consciously consider the many actions involved in the simple act of micturition.

Abnormalities of micturition

Frequency
The elderly person may not completely fill or empty the bladder and uninhibited contractions may occur during the filling and emptying, resulting in frequent desires to micturate and often the passing of only very small amounts of urine.

Urgency and precipitancy
The elderly person may have a desire to micturate and have to

do so immediately. There is often an involuntary loss of urine before this can be done.

Nocturia

There is sometimes a reversal of the normal habit and more urine is passed at night than during the day.

URINARY INCONTINENCE

Urinary incontinence occurs when there is an involuntary leakage of urine in the wrong place and at the wrong time. There are three main types:

1 stress incontinence
2 transitory incontinence
3 established incontinence.

Stress incontinence

This is an involuntary loss of urine occurring after coughing, laughing or sneezing and in which no contraction of the bladder takes place.

Cause   Bladder activity is usually normal and the fault occurs in the control of the urethral sphincter. Many suffering from stress incontinence are in the younger age group.

Treatment   In severe cases surgery may be indicated. For less severe cases pelvic floor exercises may be taught.

Transitory incontinence

This is a very common reason for admission to hospital. It also often occurs very soon after admission.

Causes:

1   Reaction to environment. Admission to a hospital or home, or moving to the home of relatives, causing anxiety, fear or even resentment, may often result in a short period of incontinence.
2   Reaction to loss of independence and identity or a move to seek attention.
3   Isolation in hospital.
4   Reaction to an acute illness. Pyrexia of unknown origin, pneumonia, urinary tract infection or a cerebrovascular acci-

dent may all result in an acute confusional state often lasting a few days only.

5 Urinary tract infection. It has been demonstrated that 20–30% of elderly people suffer from urinary tract infection and this may lead to precipitancy and often transient incontinence.

6 Faecal impaction. This is often a cause of transitory urinary incontinence and must not be overlooked. Overloading of the sigmoid colon and rectum may obstruct the bladder and impair control, leading to retention with overflow and urinary incontinence.

7 Drugs. Diuretics can often tip the balance into incontinence in a previously continent patient. Sometimes when this occurs it may be possible for the doctor to select a slower acting, gentler diuretic. Over-sedation is another common cause of incontinence, especially at night.

Established incontinence
This is present in patients who are not acutely ill and continues during their rehabilitation.

Causes:
1 Structural abnormalities of the bladder and its outlet, e.g. enlargement of the prostate gland, prolapse of the uterus and formation of cystocoele, bladder calculus or carcinoma.

2 Abnormalities affecting the nerve supply to the bladder at spinal cord level or below, e.g. cord tumours, multiple sclerosis, tabes dorsalis and subacute combined degeneration of the spinal cord.

3 Defects of the brain such as those that occur following cerebrovascular accident, cerebral tumour or cerebral arteriosclerosis. These abnormalities lead to three types of neurogenic bladder:

  a Increased bladder tone or spastic type of bladder causing urgency and decrease in volume leading to frequency when cortical control is interrupted by organic brain disease.

  b Decrease in bladder tone or atony when sensory nerve supply is damaged. Motor stimulation does not occur resulting in a large residual urine with overflow incontinence.

  c Disease or injury of the spinal cord will result in a lower centre for control. The small hypertonic bladder will act independently and frequently, resulting in the 'automatic bladder'.

Some causes of incontinence can be summarized simply in an incontinence flow chart (Fig.13).

In some hospitals incontinence clinics are now held and those patients who are fully able to co-operate may have full investigation of their bladder function with the use of sophisticated equipment, thus enabling an accurate diagnosis to be made. Urodynamic units are usually run by a urologist with a specialist nurse in attendance and are often only available on a regional basis because of the cost of the equipment.

Nursing care and the maintenance of continence

Individualized patient care has made the management of the incontinent patient easier for the nurse to handle. A careful

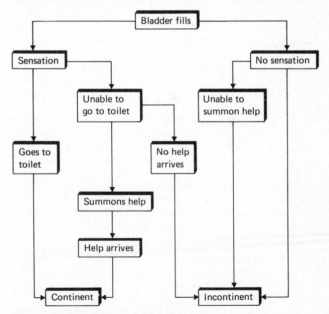

Figure 13. An incontinence flow chart.

history and assessment taken initially from the patient or relative concerned will aid the nurse's task in solving the many problems concerned with incontinence. However, investigations and treatment will be far more effective if carried out in an optimistic atmosphere where incontinence is treated as a challenge which can be overcome rather than a burden that has to be accepted. The attitude of the staff is all important—by adopting the correct approach the incidence of incontinence can be greatly reduced. Individuality, dignity and self-respect must be maintained at all times. Privacy is important to the patient and this can be achieved by drawing bed curtains and shutting the lavatory door, so the patient is not left exposed for all who are passing to see. It is important that the nurse remembers to leave the patient for only a short period of time as he may become cold and uncomfortable. Pants should be worn whenever possible, but occasionally the patient may expressly wish for these to be omitted. The lavatory should be in fairly close proximity to the patients, 10 metres being the maximum distance away if accidents are to be avoided. The door should be clearly marked or of a distinctive colour so that it is easily identifiable, and all new patients should be shown where it is situated.

A pattern of incontinence should be established and this may be done with the aid of a maintenance of continence chart (Fig. 14). Each day the patient should be allocated to a particular nurse, who should understand the importance of the task, that it is a very necessary although time-consuming job. The patient should be taken to the lavatory or commode or offered a urinal every 2 hours, and the nurse should record on the chart whether the patient is wet or dry, and whether or not he passes urine or faeces. After a few days a pattern of incontinence should evolve which will assist in planning further investigation and treatment. It may be necessary to measure the residual urine, as inefficient micturition and incomplete emptying of the bladder are increasingly common in old age.

Physical examination
1 *Mobility.* The nurse needs to observe the patient's mobility as this will give some idea whether or not the patient is able to get up out of a chair independently and reach the lavatory in a reasonable amount of time, and whether he can manage his own clothes.

MAINTENANCE OF CONTINENCE

Name: Mrs M.R.
Ward: One

DATE		DAY								MANAGEMENT	NIGHT						MANAGEMENT
month	year	8	10	12	2	4	6	8			10	12	2	4	6		
Day 1		O	+	+	+	●	+	●		2-hourly toilet	+	+	×	+	+	●	2-hourly commode
Day 2		O	●	×	+	×	+	●			●	+	O	O	+	●	
Day 3		O	+	×	O	×	O	×		2-hourly toilet	O	+	×	O	●	●	
Day 4		O	O	●	O	O	O	●			O	O	O	×	●		

Key   State of Patient
DRY   O
Incontinent of Urine   +

Result of Toileting
Passed urine in toilet   ●
Not passed urine in toilet   ×

MANAGEMENT
Preliminary check to establish pattern of micturition
Interpret chart and implement regime (2 hourly, 4 hourly, etc)
Commode by bed at night
Small drink at night with physician's advice and fluid balance chart
Correctly dressed when up

Figure 14. Maintenance of continence chart.

2 *The abdomen.* This must be examined for any signs of urinary retention and in the thin patient faecal impaction can also be observed.

3 *Perineum.* A perineal inspection should also be carried out to observe the state of the vulva or scrotum, and the condition of the skin should be recorded.

4 *Vagina.* The doctor should undertake a vaginal examination on all incontinent female patients to eliminate the possibility of a cystocoele, uterine prolapse or abnormality of the pelvic floor. Evidence of urethral tenderness and urethritis may be noted and a speculum examination may be necessary to observe the cervix and fornices.

5 *Rectum.* All patients should have a rectal examination to observe any constipation or faecal impaction. The male patient will have a rectal examination to detect the presence of an enlarged prostate gland and at the same time a bimanual examination may be carried out.

6 *Urine.* The urine should be examined for the presence of proteinuria or glycosuria which can have an effect on bladder function.

Routine investigations should also include measurement of blood urea, renal function tests, intravenous pyelogram where necessary and cystometry. Urodynamic investigations have improved understanding of bladder functioning. These include assessment of bladder function together with detrusor and sphincter activity. A fluid balance chart should be kept initially when possible, to record not only the adequate intake of fluid, but also the output of urine. When weakness of the pelvic floor is detected, effective strengthening exercises can be given by the physiotherapist.

If the incontinence is due to cerebral arteriosclerosis, a cerebrovascular accident or immobility, the patient may benefit from a period of habit training. This again must be carried out in a tranquil atmosphere and the patient allotted to a particular nurse for the day. The patient should be encouraged to go to the lavatory every 1–2 hours initially and the time span gradually increased as training progresses with the resumption of continence, and the improvement noted on the incontinence chart. This regimen should be continued at night, perhaps only disturbing the patient two or three times, and the importance explained to the night staff.

All ambulant patients should be allowed and assisted to go to the lavatory, and the less ambulant aided by the Sanichair. For those who are not able to help themselves, a commode or urinal may be used, and only on very rare occasions as a last resort, the bedpan. If used regularly, the bedpan makes difficulties later for the patient who will not have such facilities when he is discharged home or to residential accommodation. Patients balanced precariously on the bedpan in an uncomfortable position in bed, agitated at the thought of missing the pan and wetting the bed, are unlikely to be able to pass urine satisfactorily. It is essential that all patients should have access to a call system so that they may summon help when necessary.

Nocturnal incontinence

Some patients are troubled by nocturnal incontinence alone and again this must also be dealt with positively and optimistically, as it is not only demoralizing for them, but may make it difficult for their relations to have them home or for them to be accepted for residential accommodation. In order to help them overcome this problem, the patients should be encouraged to drink well during the day, and fluids should be restricted after 5 p.m. in the evening. This should be explained to the patient and the staff so that confusion and misunderstanding does not arise.

Many elderly people are accustomed to having a bucket or chamber-pot under the bed at home, and find the journey to the ward lavatory too long and difficult at night. However, this can easily be remedied by leaving a commode near the bed so that they can get in and out to this at their convenience. Some may need to be awakened and helped to the commode at regular intervals during the night, but this does not tend to disturb them unduly. There should be enough commodes on the ward to leave one by the bedside of everyone who might need it. Beds should be of adjustable height so that the patient can get in and out easily. Night sedation should be used with care, as many patients complain that they lose control at night if they have a hypnotic drug. In fact some patients benefit from an amphetamine so that they sleep lightly and wake automatically when they need to micturate.

Use of drugs

There are some drugs which have a direct effect on incontinence and should be used with care. Diuretics frequently tip the balance into incontinence in a previously continent patient, and it will be very difficult to control the incontinence if it is necessary for the patient to continue with the diuretic. A large proportion of the elderly are given diuretics to control incipient congestive cardiac failure; some may need a mild and gentle action, some need a stronger diuretic in larger doses.

Cetiprin (emepronium bromide) and Urispas (flavoxate hydrochloride) may be used to help control incontinence. These drugs have an anticholinergic effect increasing the bladder capacity by blocking the transmission of nervous impulses somewhere within the sacral reflex arc. Urispas is supplied as 100 mg tablets and the dosage is up to 2 tablets 3 times daily. Cetiprin is supplied as 100 mg tablets and the dosage is up to 200 mg three times daily and 400 mg at night. Propantheline 15–30 mg three times a day can be used to increase bladder capacity also, but it can cause dry mouth and some visual disturbances. Myotonine Chloride (bethanechol chloride) may be used in cases of urinary retention and bladder dysfunction. Di-Sipidin snuff containing antidiuretic hormone can sometimes be used at night for those with nocturnal incontinence.

Urinary tract infection

Because of the high incidence of urinary tract infection amongst the elderly, mid-stream specimens of urine should be collected from all patients on admission. The specimen should be collected in a sterile receiver, the external genitalia having previously been washed and then swabbed with Savlon solution. The specimen should be sent to the laboratory as soon as possible after it has been obtained.

The most common organisms in the infected urinary tract are the following bacteria: *Escherichia coli*, *Proteus*, and *Klebsiella*.

Treatment
- Antibiotics may be given although in some cases of recurrent urinary tract infection it is thought they are no longer effective. Some antibiotics have unpleasant side-effects causing skin rashes, nausea, diarrhoea and very rarely peripheral neuropathy.

- Fluids must be encouraged and an intake of at least 2 litres daily achieved. This is difficult as elderly women particularly are very loath to drink if incontinence is feared. A good nutritious diet should also be considered ensuring an adequate intake of calories, vitamins and protein.
- Personal hygiene should be supervised, regular baths encouraged and the patient advised to clean the perineum properly after defecation.

Pelvic floor exercises

In many units and in out-patient departments pelvic floor exercises are now taught routinely to all incontinent elderly and not just those who are suffering from stress incontinence. These exercises can be taught by the incontinence advisor or physiotherapist. There have been many beneficial results obtained after several weeks of concentrated exercise, especially amongst elderly women, and the incidence of frequency of micturition and nocturia have decreased.

Catheterization

Some patients with bladder dysfunction benefit either from a permanent indwelling catheter or from a short-term catheter released 2–4 hourly during the day in order to improve the muscle tone of the bladder.

Technique

Catheterization must be carried out with great care and aseptically in order not to introduce infection into the bladder either from the catheter or from the external genitalia. The nurse should explain carefully the procedure to the patient before she starts, giving the reasons for the necessity of an indwelling catheter. If possible the nurse should bath the patient before she begins and the patient should be in a clean bed in the recumbent position with the knees flexed, covered by a blanket. It is normally best to have another nurse present to reassure the patient and help maintain the correct position, as many elderly people find it uncomfortable and tiring. Techniques vary between different nursing schools, but a sterile technique must be strictly observed.

If the residual urine is to be measured, the patient should have emptied his bladder before the procedure commences, and the urine drained after the catheter has been placed in the bladder should be measured. Often a sterile specimen of urine is required to be sent to the laboratory for analysis. If the purpose of the catheter is to retrain the bladder muscle, it is necessary to release the catheter 2–4 hourly depending on the patient's comfort and bladder capacity. A sterile spigot should be used each time and the whole procedure carried out aseptically. Alternatively the catheter can be attached to a drainage bag and clamped and released regularly. If the catheter is withdrawn after the bladder is emptied, it should be removed gradually and the meatus swabbed. If the catheter is left in situ, it should be fixed by the use of tape to prevent any trauma occurring when the patient is moved.

Management of the catheterized patient

1 *Short-term catheterization:* A rubber catheter with an inflatable balloon can still be used, and this will last for 2–3 weeks.
2 *Long-term catheterization:* This is often necessary for the elderly and there are several different types of self-retaining catheters available which last approximately 4–6 weeks, although some can stay in situ for up to 3 months. Silicone, latex or Teflon coated catheters are all available, and trials (Kennedy, 1983) have shown that the most satisfactory are silicone and latex coated catheters and the least well tolerated Teflon.

There are two lengths now available—41 cm for males and some females, and 23 cm for females preferring to use a leg bag. The amount of water inserted in the self-retaining balloon may vary from 5 to 15 ml or 20 to 30 ml, the former now being the popular choice. In some units bladder wash-outs of normal saline or chlorhexidine may be regularly used, in others this procedure may only be carried out when debris and blockage of the catheter are a problem. The patient should be encouraged to drink an adequate amount of fluid, i.e. 2–3 litres daily.
3 *Leg bags:* The majority of elderly patients prefer to use a leg bag for draining of the catheter and this can be attached to the leg by rubber or Velcro straps under a man's trousers or a woman's stocking. The bag has a one-way valve to prevent urine leaking back into the catheter. Some patients prefer to have an ordinary drainage bag attached to a belt around the waist—a 'shepherd's sporran'. There is nothing more degrading or unpleasant for the patient or his companions than to have

to sit with a urine bag dangling from a walking-frame or chair for all to see. Patients should be taught to change and empty their own bags, using as clean a technique as possible. Used drainage bags should be burnt if possible.

There are a variety of different drainage bags available, some having easier taps to manage (Kennedy *et al.*, 1983). Some leg drainage bags can be fitted to a night bag, so they do not have to be changed every day, thus reducing cost and the likelihood of introducing infection.

Indications
There are situations when a catheter is clearly indicated:
1   When a patient is unable to go home or to an old people's home purely because he or she is incontinent.
2   When there is a pressure sore present which requires active treatment.
3   When the incontinence increases the risk of the development of a pressure sore.
4   When the patient who is occasionally incontinent requests it as opposed to the indignity of wet beds and clothing.

An elderly lady was admitted from an old people's home with a history of urinary incontinence for two years. She constantly wet the bed at night and occasionally the chair where she was sitting, and had become very unpopular with other residents because of the constant unpleasant odour.

Investigations revealed that she had a urinary tract infection which was treated with the appropriate antibiotic, and also that she had an atonic bladder with a residual urine of 1000 ml. A self-retaining catheter was inserted, spigoted and released 4-hourly, for 2 weeks, in an effort to retrain the bladder muscle. The catheter was then removed and the patient taken to the lavatory 2-hourly. The first day passed successfully, but day by day the situation deteriorated, and after 5 days and many disasters her residual urine was 800 ml. It was decided that the best solution was to leave an indwelling catheter in situ, attached to a leg bag during the day, and an ordinary drainage bag at night. The old lady was very happy, as she dreaded the incontinent episodes and learnt to change and empty her own bag. The home was happy to accept her with the catheter, and it was arranged that the home nurse would change it at regular intervals.

Aids for incontinence

There are various appliances for the incontinent patient for whom catheterization may not be practical or necessary.

For the male incontinent patient

Penile clamps   These are not often used as their siting must be exact so as to be effective without causing oedema of the penis.

Rubber urinals   These consist of a suspensory belt with a rubber sheath fitting over the penis, which is attached to a leg bag. The rubber sheath sometimes irritates the surrounding skin; however, the modern pubic pressure urinals have overcome this problem by making a short inner sleeve which fits round the pubis and base of the penis, and the outer condom remains loose.

Portex disposable urine bags   These can be attached to the scrotum by a draw-string. They are strong and light, allowing freedom of movement and causing minimal irritation.

Dribbler bags   These were introduced from Scandinavia, and consist basically of a plastic bag, of which there are two designs—the first is a plain bag and the second has a non-return valve for extra confidence. They are attached by a draw-string and very simple and easy to manage.

Sheaths   There are small sheaths of various sizes which fit tightly over the penis and held in place by a Velcro strap. The end of the sheath is then attached to a leg or ordinary drainage bag. The sheath should be changed daily and the penis thoroughly washed.

For the female incontinent patient
Aids for females are less efficient as some leakage of urine on to the skin is bound to occur.

Incontinence pants   A variety of designs are available which can be worn in conjunction with an absorbent pad which may need to be changed at regular intervals. There are a large variety now manufactured, some less dignified than others, of which a few are mentioned below. Pads and pants are only really effective if they are close fitting and comfortable. *Gellulose pads* are filled with a powder which turns to a gel when wet, thus absorbing a considerable amount of urine. They also

contain a deodorant. *Kangapants* have been designed with a
one-way fabric next to the skin and a pad on the outside in a
waterproof pocket. Attractive designs of material have been
developed which are quite acceptable for most people to wear.
Maxi-plus pants are of a different design; the pads are next to
the skin and a polythene backing prevents soiling of the
clothing. *Polyweb pads* manufactured by Smith and Nephew
are a great asset in saving laundry. They consist of four
different materials—a fine polythene net facing material, a layer
of viscose rayon staple and 12 layers of cellulose wadding
packed by a polythene sheet. They absorb quite a large amount
of fluid and help keep the patient reasonably dry.

The *Kylie sheet*, manufactured by Nicholas Products, is a
non-disposable bed sheet which can be laundered many times
without any loss of absorbency. It consists of a water-repellent,
brushed-nylon layer quilted onto an absorbing layer of rayon. It
is large and is used in conjunction with a plastic sheet because it
does not possess an impermeable backing. It has a great
absorptive capacity and the top layer is effective in keeping the
patient's skin dry.

The nurse must remember that urinary incontinence must be
viewed objectively and sympathetically and, during the investigations and subsequent management, the patients must always be treated with the utmost respect and courtesy, thus
retaining their dignity and self-respect. Patience on the part of
both patient and nurse combined with modern methods and
aids can do a great deal to reduce incontinence and alleviate the
patient's discomfort and distress.

The incontinence advisor

Much attention is now paid by the general public and health
authorities to the problems suffered by those who are incontinent. Continence advisors are now appointed to many health
authorities, these being either ward sisters involved with the
promotion of continence or nursing officers appointed specifically for that job. Their aim is to:
1   Advise incontinence sufferers and help them select the aids
available which relate most satisfactorily to their problem. They
will have firsthand knowledge of most aids on the market.

2 Instruct and educate their nurse colleagues, the medical and
paramedical staff and the general public about the problems
associated with incontinence and the promotion of continence.
3 Assist with urodynamic clinics where these are held and
become involved with research activity.

FAECAL INCONTINENCE

Faecal incontinence is far less common than urinary incontinence but it is far more difficult to tolerate and cope with,
especially in the home.

Causes
1 The most common cause and most easily treatable is faecal
impaction.
2 Diarrhoea caused by carcinoma of the colon.
3 Proctitis, colitis and diverticulitis.
4 Non-specific diarrhoea caused by poor dietary intake.
5 Rectal prolapse and haemorrhoids occurring especially in
the grand multipara due to weakness or incompetence of the
pelvic floor.

Faecal impaction

The elderly frequently become obsessed with their bowels and
are distressed if they have not passed one loose motion every
day. As a result they tend to take various favourite purgatives
which may have been in use since childhood. This may have
been their practice for some years, with the result that the colon
no longer reacts to stimulation and becomes over-distended.
Eventually constant stretching of the rectum and pelvic colon
produces weakness and lack of tone of the muscular wall. The
bulk of faecal mass tends to be small and hard, thus failing to
stimulate reflex action in the rectum, which anyway is frequently diminished in later life.

Causes of faecal impaction
1 Constipation in a person confined to bed.
2 Dehydration from diminished fluid intake.
3 Use of high residue food substances.
4 Use of bulk laxatives and analgesics such as codeine.

The large bowel becomes overloaded and the faecal mass becomes dry and hard, causing loss of sphincter control. Eventually hard faeces in the rectum act as an irritant to the mucosal lining and the mucus secreted dissolves some of the faecal mass, causing a little liquid stool to be excreted in the form of spurious diarrhoea.

Signs and symptoms
1   Faecal impaction is usually suspected from soiling of the patient's underwear or sheets.
2   There is the typical stale offensive smell of faecal matter.
3   On abdominal examination, faecal masses may be seen in thin patients.
4   On rectal examination, faecal masses may be felt by indentation.
5   Plain X-ray of the abdomen may reveal faecal masses especially when high impaction is suspected.

Treatment
- The stool should be softened by the use of a stool softener such as Dioctyl-Medo or danthron. These are a combination of a wetting agent and a mild peristaltic stimulant which, given at night, may also prevent further impaction.
- Daily enemas should be given until the result of the enema is the return of fluid free from faecal matter.
- Initially it may be necessary to do a digital removal of the stool if it is very hard, and this should only be done by an experienced nurse or doctor.
- Those patients who are unable to tolerate an enema may be given four to five glycerol suppositories.

Prevention
Once the bowel is empty, constipation should be prevented in the following ways:
- Faulty dietary habits should be corrected by increasing intake of vitamins and roughage. Bran should be added to the diet as fibre is a safe and effective remedy for constipation. It can be added to cereals and soups, and the use of wholemeal bread should be recommended. Consumption of fruit should also be encouraged, not only fresh oranges and apples but also prunes and rhubarb.
- The fluid intake of the elderly is often very low, and extra drinks of tea and fruit juice should be offered frequently.

- Faulty toilet habits and impaired mental awareness may be improved with a period of training.

Very occasionally faecal impaction causes sub-acute intestinal obstruction, and the patient with a ball of faeces as large as a melon in the caecal region has been known to undergo a laparotomy to relieve the obstruction.

Complications of faecal impaction

1 Overloading of the sigmoid colon and rectum in impaction may obstruct the bladder and impair control, perhaps leading to retention with overflow and urinary incontinence.

2 Diverticulosis and diverticulitis may be caused and aggravated by constipation and impaction. Small diverticula are found in 5–10% of persons over middle age, most commonly in the pelvic colon. Diverticulosis is symptomless. If the openings in the diverticulae become narrow, faecal material may stagnate in the pouches and infection occur, giving rise to symptoms and an acute form of the disease known as diverticulitis, with all its complications.

Inflammatory changes lead to thickening of the affected area of the colon which may be adherent to the surrounding structures causing fistulae, perforation or haemorrhage. The disease may flare up for periods over many years causing abdominal pain, generally left-sided and associated with defecation. Occasionally a mass is felt in the left iliac fossa and may be confused with a carcinoma. Diagnosis is made by sigmoidoscopy and barium enema. Treatment is to give a well-balanced diet that is non-irritating and yet prevents constipation occurring. Bulk-producing aperients such as Isogel (ispaghula husk) may be used.

Treatment of other forms of diarrhoea

- *Non-specific diarrhoea* will be improved by giving a well balanced diet and regular doses of kaolin. *Proctitis* and *colitis* may be treated with an anti-inflammatory drug or a bulk maker. Occasionally it may be necessary to give a short course of oral steroids or a retention enema containing steroids.
- *Rectal prolapse* may occur, causing loss of sphincter control and incontinence. There is weakness of the muscles of the pelvic floor as the result of chronic constipation and the

rectal wall protrudes through the anus. Surgical treatment may be necessary with the insertion of a ring or tantalum wire round the anus. Great care must be exercised to ensure that faecal impaction does not follow surgery.

- *Neuromuscular inco-ordination of the anal sphincter* has been successfully treated by a battery-operated pulsator. Severe cerebral damage due to a cerebrovascular accident or cerebral arteriosclerosis will produce lack of cortical control leading to faecal incontinence, but the patient may respond to the regular use of suppositories or enemas.

The use of enemas

A fully comprehensive explanation must be given to the patient by the nurse before the procedure is begun. The windows are closed and the patient laid on the bed on his left side with his knees drawn up, the bed having been well protected with a disposable draw-sheet and incontinence pads. A commode should be placed near the bedside. After the enema has been given it may take some considerable time for full evacuation to take place. The patient should be seated in a comfortable position on the commode or lavatory, ensuring that he is quite warm. When the procedure is completed, the patient usually appreciates a warm bath.

There are a variety of enemas on the market, of which the most commonly used are:

1 *Soap enema or enema saponis.* This is made from soft soap and water. It is given at 37.5°C and the elderly patient usually tolerates 250–300 ml. This is often the most effective and efficient enema.

2 *Disposable phosphate enema.* This comes in a pack and should be warmed in a bowl of water before being given. It is more effective if a rectal tube is placed on the end so it can be inserted fairly high up into the rectum.

3 *Glycerol enema.* This is a more gentle and lubricating enema. About 60 ml of glycerol is added to 200 ml of warm water and run in very slowly.

4 *Olive oil retention enema.* In cases of severe impaction where the patient is fit, an olive oil enema may be given to be retained overnight. 100–200 ml of warm oil is slowly run into the rectum and the bed is tipped on blocks for the night. This is followed by an enema saponis the next morning.

5 *Micralax and dioctyl enemas.* These are much smaller in volume and not as effective, but are less traumatic.

6 *Glycerol, bisacodyl and Beogex suppositories.* These may be given to relieve simple constipation and to the more frail patients.

In conclusion it must be said that on the whole urinary incontinence is controllable and faecal incontinence preventable. The success of the treatment will depend very largely upon the preparation of the individual care plan, the atmosphere within the ward and the optimistic attitude of the staff.

References

Kennedy, A.P. (1983) Incontinence advice—long term catheterization. *Nursing Times* (April).

Kennedy, A.P., Brocklehurst, J.C. & Faragher, B. (1983) A comparison of 10 urinary drainage bags. *Nursing Times* (Aug.)

Wade, B., Sawyer, L. & Bell, J. (1983) *Dependency with Dignity*. London: Bedford Square Press.

Wells, T.J. (1980) *Problems in Geriatric Nursing Care.* Edinburgh: Churchill Livingstone.

Further reading

Incontinence Handbook (1983) Thames Valley Medical.

Mandelstam, D. (1980) *Incontinence and its Management.* London: Croom Helm.

The Problems of Promoting Continence (1982) London: Rcn and Squibb Surgicare Ltd.

7
Pressure Sores and their Prevention

Prevention of pressure sores is a dominant feature in the nursing care of the elderly whether at home or in hospital. It is a growing problem, as has been indicated by Norton *et al.* (1975), whose calculations show that the evidence of sores is considerably higher in the over 70 and 80 age groups. The development of a pressure sore not only increases the time that the elderly are treated in hospital but also increases the amount of nursing care required and the cost to the National Health Service. A survey done by Norton, Mclaren and Exton-Smith in 1962 showed that the mortality rate was five times as great in those who developed sores and the length of stay in hospital was much longer, although it must be remembered that those who had pressure sores were generally more debilitated than those who did not. The cost to the health service is approximately £100 million (Torrance, 1983) and this may well increase. Development of sores interferes considerably with the patient's rehabilitation and can be a contributory cause of death. A sore can form within a day and take months to heal, so the prevention and treatment are extremely important and deserve much consideration. The onus falls mainly on the nursing staff, with help and advice from the physiotherapist and medical staff.

On admission to hospital or on commencement of treatment for a patient at home, the nurse will take a nursing history and thoroughly examine the patient, looking particularly for any signs of sores. She will make an assessment, and may be helped in this by making use of a simple scoring system whereby the patient's mental and physical condition is assessed. This system was devised by Doreen Norton and others (1962) and has been widely used since. A high score will reveal a fairly able, alert and ambulant patient, and a low score a debilitated, confused and incontinent patient who is greatly at risk. This system will

also identify those borderline cases who need constant attention. The system should be reviewed weekly and incorporated
into the regular evaluation to assess those who deteriorate and
those who improve. It can help in the formation of the care
plan, indicating those who need intensive care, those who need
intermediate care and those who require supervision only. The
type of care indicated in the care plan as to treatment of existing
sores and use of pressure-relieving devices will depend upon the
comfort of the patient, the preference of the nursing staff and
the equipment available. Some methods will be discussed later
in this chapter.

Types of sores

The common sites of sores when the patient is recumbent are
shoulders, elbows, buttocks and heels (Fig. 15). In the severely
debilitated patient, sores can also develop on the ears and back
of the head.

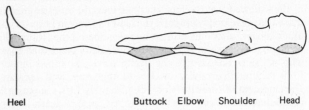

Heel   Buttock Elbow Shoulder Head

Figure 15. Common sites of pressure sores.

There are four main types of sores:
1   Deep sores due to *sustained pressure*, i.e. from sitting or lying
on a hard surface for a length of time, e.g. theatre, X-ray
trolley, casualty department, paraplegic patients sitting in a
chair or lying in bed unable to move.
2   Sores due to a *shearing force* when two surfaces slide against
each other, in which the exterior skin is fixed but the underlying fascia is damaged, e.g. due to bad positioning in bed or in
a chair.
3   Superficial sores due to *friction*, e.g. when a patient is
dragged up the bed or in a chair, causing friction between the
bedclothes and the skin. These can be very painful.
4   Superficial sores due to *constant moisture*, as occurs for

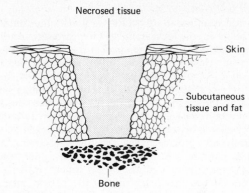

Figure 16. Deep sore.

example in the incontinent patient or when there is leakage from a catheter.

The majority of the sores develop within the first two weeks of the patient's stay in hospital, and thus the early days after admission seem to be the time when patients are particularly at risk, hence the necessity for intensive observation and prophylaxis by the nursing staff.

Prevention

The nurse must always aim to prevent these sores, so prevention will be considered before treatment of established sores. As the main cause of tissue damage is sustained pressure, the main object of prevention is to relieve pressure.

The two main aetiological factors of poor general condition and immobility are often interrelated. Heart and respiratory disease are liable to increase risk due to poor circulation. Neurological diseases interfere with the nerve supply to the skin and muscle. Incidence is also high in cerebral arteriosclerosis and malignant disease whereas it is low in musculoskeletal disease.

The patient is greatly at risk if he suffers from drowsiness due to over-sedation, poor nutrition, anaemia or urinary, faecal or double incontinence. If some of these conditions are present, help and advice must be sought from the physician.

Relief of pressure

Rest in bed resulting in immobility is usually the commonest complication in the development of a pressure sore, and therefore whenever possible the patient must be encouraged to be ambulant. However, in those for whom bedrest is essential or who have to spend long periods of time in bed, regular turning is essential, the length of time depending on the condition of the patient. Primarily, those patients who are in bed should be turned 2-hourly. Those who have no sores but are at risk should be turned systematically from right lateral to left lateral and, provided they are fully conscious, to the recumbent position. The semi-prone position is not generally tolerated nor comfortable for the elderly patient. In some cases where the skin is extremely fragile, the patient may need turning as often as hourly, but for the fitter patient who is able to move unaided, 4-hourly turning may be adequate. The skin should be washed if the patient is incontinent or sweating, and applications of creams and powders vary according to the individual ward sister's preference. Early rehabilitation should be aimed at and this may also help to control some incontinence. The underlying causes of the patient's immobility must be investigated and where possible treated by the medical staff, so that the length of stay in bed is reduced to a minimum, and immobility corrected as soon as possible. Devices which can be used for relief of pressure will be discussed later.

Sedation

Using apparatus to record bodily movements during sleep, it has been shown that reduced mobility is directly related to the incidence of pressure sores. Therefore, whenever possible very light sedation, or better still no sedation at all, should be used, especially at night. Any over-sedation should be noted and reported by the nurse, and the doctor should be encouraged to reduce the sedation wherever possible.

Nutrition

A well-balanced diet should be given, with specific attention being given to adequate protein and vitamins. The diet may be complemented with high-protein drinks such as supplemented milk shakes. High potency vitamin supplements are frequently indicated. Fluids should be encouraged—daily intake should be two litres.

Anaemia
Anaemia should be corrected and in some cases blood transfusion may be necessary, although if the cause of the anaemia is nutritional or due to malabsorption, the patient will respond to intramuscular iron. It may also be necessary to give oral folic acid and intramuscular cyanocobalamin.

Incontinence
Urinary incontinence should be treated positively and if no improvement is noted following the investigation of the cause and the introduction of training regimens, a catheter may be considered while the patient is particularly prone to develop a sore. Faecal incontinence should be treated and may nearly always be prevented (see chapter 6).

Skin care
Good skin care should be initiated by the nurse. The areas at risk should be washed with soap and water two or three times daily and more often when incontinence is a problem. The natural oil is lost from superficial layers of skin through frequent washing with soap and water, on account of the alkaline content of the soap, and the application of zinc and castor oil cream can help to replace the oil in the incontinent patient. Silicone creams may also be useful as barrier creams to protect the skin. However, some barrier creams can cause irritation and allergies, so they should be used with caution. The bed sheet should be free of rucks, crumbs and creases which irritate the skin. Where possible plastic sheeting and incontinence pads should not be used as these too can irritate the skin.

Those patients at risk must be carefully examined daily and any signs of redness or blisters noted and dealt with accordingly. There are a large range of preparations for local application to the pressure sore, and this is itself indicative of the lack of knowledge regarding the best preparation. The real danger, irrespective of their individual merits, is reliance on these preparations to the exclusion of knowledge of the patient's condition and the relief of or reduction of pressure.

Pressure relieving equipment
This varies from very simple, inexpensive devices to very sophisticated, costly pieces of equipment, as follows:

a   The *bed cradle* is a very necessary piece of equipment to relieve pressure in the heels.

b   *Heel and elbow pads* may also be used, e.g. the Parapad (Seton), which is a fleece-lined Tubigrip, or the Spenco heel pad, which is based on silicone padding.

c   *Foam* is widely used nowadays, and the Lennard pad (Fig. 17), or 'cheese' as it is commonly called, has been developed by Professor Brocklehurst for the relief of pressure on the heels. It can be secured in the bed by a draw-sheet, and constant surveillance must be maintained to ensure that, when the patient moves, the wedge is also moved. Foam pads are also useful for relieving pressure between the knees and occasionally for protecting heels and elbows, although the nurse must remove them frequently to check that the skin remains in good condition.

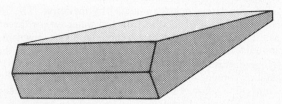

Figure 17. Lennard pad.

d   *Cushions.* There are a variety of cushions now on the market for use in chairs and wheelchairs. Foam rings may be useful for some patients. The Cubex cushion is filled with polystyrene beads which alter the pressure with the slightest movement—it is used regularly by airline pilots! The compressed sponge foam cushion allows the patient to sit for long periods with a reduction of pressure over bony prominences. Such cushions are particularly useful for allowing those patients who have a tendency to develop a sore or who already have an early sore to sit in a chair. The Spenco cushion is filled with silicone padding.

e   *The sheepskin and synthetic fleece.* These are widely used in the bed, in the chair, and for heels. The natural spring of the wool helps to relieve pressure on the areas of the body in contact with it, the fibres distributing the weight of the patient over a large area and providing an air circulation

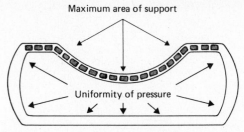

Maximum area of support

Uniformity of pressure

No counter pressure effect from **compressed** sponge foam

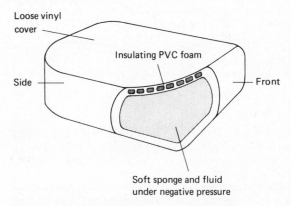

Loose vinyl cover

Insulating PVC foam

Side

Front

Soft sponge and fluid under negative pressure

Figure 18. Compressed sponge foam cushion.

there, and this also helps to keep the skin dry. Since sheepskin can absorb water up to one third of its dry weight without feeling wet, even patients who perspire freely can benefit from its use. It also prevents friction in the sacral area or wherever else it is used.

f   *Mattresses and beds.* The large cell ripple mattress consists of plastic tubes 10 cm (4 in) in diameter which are alternately filled with air pumped electrically in 10-minute cycles. The tubes may be removed in the appropriate place if the patient has a pressure sore. The small cell ripple mattress has proved useful for very light patients only and is now little used. These mattresses should be used early enough and kept in good order. The foam mattress will

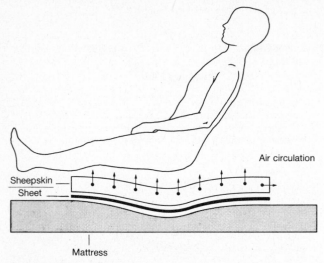

Figure 19. The sheepskin.

reduce tension if used without a cover, but it is not often practical. The Spenco mattress has silicone padding which prevents abrasive injury. It is comfortable and gives light relief of pressure.

The *net suspension bed* is an effective yet fairly inexpensive piece of equipment used in the healing and prevention of pressure sores. It can be attached to most bedsteads. The patient is suspended in a nylon mesh net, which enables him to be turned without any direct physical effort from either the patient or the nurse. The advantages of the net bed are the equal distribution of weight over the underside of the body and circulation of air, keeping the temperature cool and reducing humidity. It is only really effective in treating patients in the recumbent position. It does not prevent shearing stress.

The *water bed* consists of a tough, thin, flexible membrane for the mattress supported by a fibreglass tank on a mobile steel structure. The relief of pressure in a controlled bed depends on the degree of flotation. Difficulty is experienced in lifting and nursing patients. It has a limited use and is not liked by some patients.

Treatment

The aim of the nurse here is to promote healing and prevent infection. The patient generally needs to be nursed in bed, and rapid healing is desirable so that mobilization is not long delayed. When his general condition improves it may be possible to allow the patient to sit out for short periods, providing no pressure is exerted on the affected area. It should be remembered that nurses, through a false impression of security, may neglect those severely incapacitated patients confined most of the day to a chair. They should have the pressure removed from the sacral area for a few minutes every half hour.

Factors necessary for healing to take place:
1   The area needs to be free of necrotic material. This can be removed by a de-sloughing agent such as Aserbine or Eusol. Ultraviolet light may help de-sloughing of necrotic tissue and stimulation of the growth of granulation tissue.
2   The surrounding tissue needs to be healthy and to have a good blood supply. Ultrasound has been found to promote healing.

Factors preventing healing:
1   Presence of infection, which may have to be treated with antibiotics.
2   Defective oxygenation of the area due to a poor blood supply.
3   Presence of oedema.
4   Continued trauma.
5   Development of a sinus leading to infection of underlying bones. This may have to be opened and drained.

In general the patient with a sacral sore should be nursed in bed off the sore. If it is superficial it should be kept dry, but may respond well to a daily saline bath. If the patient does sit out of bed, a sheepskin may be used as this relieves friction. If the sore is deep it is essential to keep the area clean and moist and the dressing applied needs to reflect this. If drainage is necessary the dressing needs to be changed easily but in some cases semi-permeable dressing may be used such as Opsite. This is a semi-permeable adhesive polyurethane membrane which retains the wound exudate but does not allow infection to enter, thus creating a suitable environment for healing to take place. This dressing should not be changed except when infection is present until healing has taken place.

If a heel sore is being treated, pressure should be removed from the bedclothes by use of a cradle and from the bed by use of a wedge. The patient may sit out but the affected foot should be elevated so as to reduce oedema and improve circulation. Walking should be encouraged if possible.

The general health of a patient must be considered, as sores obviously do not usually occur in those who are healthy and well nourished. Much protein is lost through the established sore and protein is the only foodstuff containing nitrogen which is vital for producing new tissues and replacing waste. A negative nitrogen balance can be avoided by high protein feeding and the use of anabolic agents like Deca-Durabolin (nandrolone). Therefore a high protein diet should be given, which should also be rich in vitamins, especially vitamin C, sometimes given direct to the patient in the form of ascorbic acid.

If the patient is unable to eat normally, a liquid diet should be given reinforced with Casilan and high protein drinks. It may be necessary to pass a nasogastric tube and temporarily feed the patient in this way. Fluids should be encouraged, with at least 2 litres per day being the aim of the nurse.

Antibiotics need rarely be used except when plastic surgery is indicated, or in the case of a diabetic patient, where active and urgent measures need to be taken to prevent extension of the sore. Local antibiotics do not usually prove effective. Some centres have found the application of various forms of syrups and sugars efficient in promoting healing. Obviously prevention of incontinence is essential. Catheterization is indicated if the patient is incontinent of urine, as occasional incontinence especially at night can have a very harmful effect on the cleaning and healing processes. Faecal incontinence must also be controlled.

The complications of pressure sores are many and serious, reinforcing the thesis that prevention is better than cure. Cellulitis, venous thrombosis and emboli may all occur with resulting swelling, inflammation and pain. Bacteraemia may develop which may eventually lead to pyelonephritis, arthritis, meningitis and endocarditis, all of which may have very serious complications. Loss of protein and electrolyte imbalance may also occur, and death of the patient may be the eventual outcome of a severe or extensive pressure sore.

References

Norton, D., Mclaren, R. & Exton-Smith, A.N. (1962) *An Investigation of Geriatric Nursing Problems in Hospital.* Edinburgh: Churchill Livingstone (reissued 1975).

Torrance, C. (1983) *Pressure Sores: Aetiology, Treatment and Prevention.* London: Croom Helm.

Further reading

Barton, A. & Barton, M. (1981) *The Management and Prevention of Pressure Sores.* London: Faber & Faber.

David, J.A., Chapman, R.G., Chapman, E.J. & Lockett, B. (1984) Survey of prescribed nursing treatment for patients with established pressure sores. Paper presented at WENR/Rcn international conference 11–13 April. (Available from the Nursing Practice Research Unit, Northwick Park.)

Nursing—The Add-on Journal of Clinical Nursing. Jan 1984—Pressure Sores.

Walker, K.A. (1971) *Pressure Sores: Prevention and Treatment.* London: Butterworths.

8
Nutrition

Good nutrition throughout a person's life has a direct bearing on his health in old age, and there is a direct relationship between poor eating habits earlier in life and chronic disease in later life. As Cheyne said in 1725 'most of all chronic diseases, the infirmities of old age and the short period of the lives of Englishmen are owing to repletion'. Most old people require less calories as their basal metabolic rate and physical activity decrease, but require as much, if not more, basic nutrients such as protein, minerals and vitamins.

Studies carried out among the elderly have shown that this section of the population represents the largest single group vulnerable to malnutrition. Elderly house-bound people have been found to have nutrient intakes which are substantially lower than those of active people of comparable age. Eating in institutions too can have its disadvantages—food cooked in bulk can lack some vital nutrients and often appears unappetizing to the consumer.

The energy value of foods is measured in heat units—kilojoules (kJ)—which provides an assessment of the amounts of food required by different people in accordance with their age, build and occupation. The chief broad groups of foods will provide the following values in kilojoules:

1 g carbohydrate (as glucose)	16 kJ
1 g fat	39 kJ
1 g protein	17 kJ

The normal energy requirements of an elderly man upon retirement are approximately 9600 kJ per day and should stay at this level as long as he remains active; the basal requirements may be only 6000 kJ. For women the requirement is 6000–8500 kJ and the basal requirement 5500 kJ.

The recommended daily intakes are as follows:

Women	55–57 years	Energy 8600 kJ	Protein 53 g
	75+ years	Energy 8000 kJ	Protein 53 g
Men	67–75 years	Energy 9800 kJ	Protein 63 g
	75+ years	Energy 8800 kJ	Protein 63 g

CARBOHYDRATES

These are sugars and starches and are composed of carbon, hydrogen and oxygen only. They are transported in the bloodstream and are converted into carbon dioxide and water, releasing some energy as heat, the remainder being stored in the form of glycogen in the liver and cells, being used as necessary to maintain a chemical balance and for physical activity. A certain concentration of glucose is maintained in the blood by the liver and varies between 5 and 10 mmol/litre.

Sources: fruit, sugar, potatoes, flour, bread, rice.

Excess causes obesity and digestive disorders.

Deficiency can lead to ketosis, when fat is used for the production of energy to a greater extent than normal. The majority of elderly people have a high intake of carbohydrates as they are found in the less expensive forms of food and need little preparation.

Cellulose consists of large molecules of carbohydrate which cannot be split and pass unaltered through the alimentary tract. Cellulose is contained in fruit and vegetables and, since they stimulate peristalsis of the bowel, these help to establish regular bowel habits.

FAT

Although fat has the same constituents as glucose (i.e. carbon, hydrogen and oxygen), it can release more energy per unit weight. Any excess fat is stored in the fat deposits in the body, mainly subcutaneously and around the abdominal organs. Fat is a component of cell membranes and is particularly important with regard to the cells of the nervous system.

Sources: butter, meat, milk, some fish, lard, vegetable oils and nut oils when converted into margarine.

There is some relation between fats and arterial disease in which fatty materials are deposited in the arterial walls, but no absolute recommendation about diets in this respect seems justifiable for this age group. However, it is important in early years to reduce the incidence of cerebrovascular disease, myocardial infarction, peripheral vascular disease and diabetes mellitus, by exercising care with the quantity of fats consumed.

PROTEIN

Protein is a principal constituent of every living cell. Protein is composed of carbon, hydrogen, oxygen and nitrogen, and is the only food source of nitrogen for the body. It consists of amino acids, of which there are known to be 24. Of these, 10 are considered to be *essential* in the adult (i.e. they cannot be synthesized in the body in sufficient amounts and need to be obtained in the diet).

Some protein is lost to the body during metabolism and amino acids from the diet are necessary for replacement. Amino acids are required by the tissues for the production of enzymes, hormones, haemoglobin and antibodies. Protein is also a source of energy.

Sources: animal protein such as meat, fish, cheese, eggs and milk; vegetable protein such as green peas, lentils, peanuts, baked beans.

Studies have shown that women with high protein intake enjoy better health than those with low intake. The daily intake should not fall with age and should be 1 g/kg of body weight per day. There is an increased need in debilitating illness and conditions with excessive loss, e.g. severe pressures sores; this may be assisted by the use of anabolic steroids.

Protein, particularly meat, is an expensive form of food and therefore not always eaten in sufficient quantities. Cheese and milk are widely consumed. Bread contains a certain amount of protein, and many elderly people obtain as much as 20% of their protein from this source. Eggs are also an excellent and cheap form of protein.

VITAMINS

Fat-soluble vitamins

Vitamin A
This is essential for normal vision and maintains the epithelial tissue of the body.

Sources: meat, fish, fish oils, butter, cheese.

Deficiency, rarely seen in the elderly, results in night-blindness and infections of the mucous membranes.

Vitamin K
This is essential for the formation of prothrombin in the liver, which is required for the clotting of blood.

Source: green vegetables.

Deficiency: no evidence in the elderly except in obstructive jaundice when lack of bile salts will impair absorption.

Vitamin D
This increases the absorption of calcium and phosphorus from the digestive tract and promotes the deposition on the bone. Much of the body's requirement is met by synthesis in the skin by ultraviolet light in the form of sunlight, which is often missed by the elderly.

Source: eggs, fish, margarine, sunlight.

Deficiency: in children—rickets; in the elderly—a) evidence of osteomalacia which may be symptomless unless a fracture occurs, b) general muscle weakness, waddling gait, difficulty climbing stairs, low back pain, c) stiffness and bone tenderness, d) malabsorption, e) liver and kidney disease.

Water-soluble vitamins

Vitamin B
This is a complex of different vitamins: thiamine (B_1), riboflavin (B_2), niacin, pyridoxine (B_6), pantothenic acid, biotin, folic acid and cyanocobalamin (B_{12}).

Thiamine This constitutes part of an enzyme system concerned in the metabolism of carbohydrate.

Source: wholemeal flour and bread, liver.

Deficiency: a) Principal cause of beriberi, which occurs among people whose staple food is polished rice, since thiamine is found in the discarded husks of rice. Causes polyneuritis, which involves the legs and feet, and results in pain, weakness and inability to co-ordinate. b) Acute confusional states and neuritis among the elderly.

Riboflavin   This is essential for tissue oxidation.

Source: milk, liver, kidneys, heart, egg yolk.

Deficiency results in glossitis and dermatitis round the mouth, nose, vulva and scrotum. Deficiency is rare in this country.

Niacin or nicotinic acid   This has similar action to riboflavin.

Source: yeast, wholemeal bread, liver, meat.

Deficiency, along with other vitamins of the B complex, causes pellagra. Reddish-brown areas appear on the skin, especially the neck, face and hands. Dermatitis, diarrhoea and dementia may also occur.

Pyridoxine   This has an important action in amino acid metabolism.

Source: yeast, liver, wheat, corn.

Deficiency leads to mental confusion, depression and dermatitis.

Cyanocobalamin   This is the extrinsic factor necessary for normal red cell maturation, but it cannot be absorbed without the intrinsic factor present in gastric secretions.

Source: liver, kidney, heart, fish, cheese, eggs.

Deficiency: Found in the elderly who lack the intrinsic factor necessary for absorption due to impairment of gastric secretions. The patient develops Addisonian or pernicious anaemia, named after Addison of Guy's Hospital who described the condition in 1855. The onset is gradual, with symptoms not presenting until the haemoglobin is below 6 g/dl. Symptoms and signs are breathlessness, weakness, swollen ankles, and a lemon or yellow tint to the skin. Treatment is by intramuscular injections of cyanocobalamin, daily initially and eventually 3-monthly for the rest of the patient's life.

Subacute combined degeneration of the spinal cord is closely associated with Addisonian anaemia. The patient complains of numbness in the feet and fingers, weakness and unsteadiness when walking. The treatment is similar to that of Addisonian anaemia, but they cyanocobalamin is given more frequently initially and in larger doses.

Folic acid   This, like cyanocobalamin, is necessary for the development of red blood corpuscles and maturation of the nuclei.

Source: green leafy vegetables.

Deficiency occurs when the elderly have disorders of the gastrointestinal tract giving rise to malabsorption. It may be replaced in oral form.

Vitamin C

This is necessary for the formation of red cells and the absorption of iron. It is also required for the metabolism of amino acids, and the formation of collagen in connective tissue, and is thus necessary for sound healing of wounds.

Vitamin C is the most easily destroyed vitamin, although it is less easily destroyed in dried foods. In homes and hospitals where there is bulk cooking and vegetables tend to be cooked for too long and then kept warm for several hours before delivering them to the patient, there is a real risk of vitamin C deficiency. The most common vegetables are potatoes and cabbage. To retain the maximum amount of vitamin C the vegetables should be cooked unpeeled if possible and in large pieces so that water-soluble nutrients are not lost through the cut surfaces. As little water as possible should be used and they should be cooked for the shortest possible time and served immediately. Ascorbic acid is easily destroyed by heat and exposure to light.

Source: citrus fruit such as oranges, lemons, grapefruit; tomatoes; leafy vegetables; soft fruits such as blackcurrants, gooseberries, raspberries, strawberries. Potatoes have a small, but important, amount as they are the staple food of many who cannot afford the more expensive fruit.

Deficiency causes weakness, irritability, decreased resistance to infection and pains in the limbs and joints. Prolonged deficiency causes scurvy, in which there are multiple haemorrhages, swollen painful gums, haemorrhages into the joints and degenerative changes of the bones.

Mr X., aged 82, was admitted from home thought to be deficient in vitamin C. His wife had died 2 years previously, and although he had managed well at first, he had gradually sunk into a state of apathy and was existing on tinned rice pudding. He was edentulous but his gums appeared swollen; he was very irritable and obstreperous at times; he had a few petechial haemorrhages and unhealed varicose ulcers on both legs which were heavily infected and neglected. Mr X. commenced large doses of ascorbic acid, 100 g three times daily; he was also given a nutritious but soft diet, rich in protein, and wherever possible fresh fruit. The infections of his legs were treated and slowly the ulcers began to heal. Several months later Mr X. was fit enough to leave hospital and he agreed reluctantly to leave his home and live in council residential accommodation. He never would agree to see a dentist!

MINERALS

Calcium

This is the mineral which occurs in the greatest amount in the body and is the structural component of bone. It is absorbed from the alimentary tract with the aid of vitamin D.

Source: milk and cheese are the main sources. Milk has a high content, is easily available, relatively inexpensive and a staple food.

Deficiency gives rise to osteoporosis, which is a common disorder in elderly persons, especially woman. There is a reduction of the bone mass with a change in the constitution. The bones become radiologically less dense and clinically more brittle. Pain is symptomatic. There is sometimes kyphosis and loss of height but many patients also have a compression fracture of the vertebral bodies. Treatment and progress are slow. Calcium can be given orally and can be enhanced by anabolic steroids, e.g. Durabolin (nandrolone). Spinal support may be helpful and necessary.

Iron

Iron is necessary for the formation of haemoglobin, which is a constituent of the red blood cells. Haemogobin is responsible for the transportation of oxygen and carbon dioxide between the lungs and the tissues. Only a small quantity of iron is absorbed from food and this is facilitated by ascorbic acid and possibly hydrochloric acid, as iron deficiency is usually present when there is achlorhydria (absence of hydrochloric acid in the stomach). Achlorhydria is common in old age, so this might explain the malabsorption of iron resulting in iron deficiency anaemia. Iron absorption is also enhanced by the presence of protein. Eggs may appear to be a good source of iron, but it has been found that the iron in egg is bound to phosphates and may not be available to the body. Generally about 5–10% of iron in the diet is absorbed but if someone is anaemic then the absorption of iron will be enhanced.

The elderly also tend to suffer from minor gastrointestinal disorders such as haemorrhoids, hiatus hernia and gastric ulcerations with chronic loss of blood.

It has been found difficult to maintain the iron content of hospital diets at an acceptable level, so it must be much more difficult for the elderly living alone on restricted incomes.

Source: meat, especially liver, eggs, green leafy vegetables, fish, wholemeal flour and bread.

CEREAL FIBRE

Bran is now thought to be an important constituent of the diet because of its promoting normal bowel function. Bran consumed in earlier life may help prevent bowel complications in old age. Many elderly suffer from diverticular disease and chronic constipation, and the addition of bran to the diet can help ease these problems.

Source: pure bran, wholemeal flour, some cereals.

FLUID REQUIREMENTS

The elderly person requires approximately 2 litres of liquid every 24 hours, and this should be increased if fever, sweating, polyuria or dehydration are present. If eating normally, the patient will ingest 1 litre of fluid in his food but if not 2 litres must be provided in fluids.

Frequently it is very difficult to persuade elderly patients to drink this amount, especially women who do not wish to be disturbed at night or who fear to wet the bed. Many find it a great effort to drink when ill, and some have difficulty in swallowing. Restriction of fluid can lead to chronic constipation. Surveys carried out on the elderly in hospital and in community homes reveal that they often drink much less than 2 litres per day. Enticing fluids should be offered frequently. There are now a wide variety of drinks on the market which should cater for every taste.

MALNUTRITION

Causes of malnutrition

The most common cause of malnutrition is inadequate diet, for which there are a variety of causes:

1   The elderly person may live alone, thus having no incentive to cook adequate meals.

2   The elderly person may live alone and have difficulty shopping, cooking, and preparing food because of physical disability, e.g. those with arthritis, parkinsonism and following a cerebrovascular accident. Some elderly people are not supplied with the necessary tools to assist them when cooking.

3   The elderly man, living alone following the death of his wife, may find he cannot manage to feed himself adequately.

4   Depression in the elderly may cause loss of appetite leading to a general deterioration and malnutrition.

5   The elderly person living on a very small income cannot afford the correct foods and is unaware of the financial benefits available within the Welfare State. The more desirable foods are not only more expensive, but take more time and trouble to cook as well as being perishable. This is all the more pertinent with the rising cost of living.

6   Disorders of digestion and ill fitting dentures may result in an inadequate dietary intake.

7   Lack of knowledge of the value of food and the necessary dietary intake.

8   Excessive use of alcohol.

9   The ever-increasing use of convenience foods, which often lack essential nutrients.

People with the above problems may benefit from various facilities available to help them, such as:

1   Luncheon Clubs, usually run by the Women's Royal Voluntary Service once or twice a week, where a balanced meal can be enjoyed in a congenial atmosphere.

2   A day club or day centre usually run by Age Concern in a town, again where good food can be enjoyed in good company, and some people may be able to attend several times a week. This may help to correct the inadequate diet received at home.

3   Meals-on-wheels, prepared and delivered by the Women's Royal Voluntary Service, are provided 2, 3 or 5 times a week and help to provide a nutritious meal on these occasions, thus

supplementing an otherwise inadequate diet.

4   The home help service, organized by the social services department of the local authority, aims to provide someone to cook a meal regularly in the elderly person's home where this is necessary. This person will also shop and thus see that there is food in the house in the interim period.

5   Investigation and treatment of the digestive disorder may be necessary, and a visit to the dentist may be advised. Those who have difficulty with equipment may benefit from a visit from the occupational therapist.

6   Advice on food may be given at the day centre.

Obesity

Obesity is a more common disease than undernutrition, especially among women. Causes include:

1   Ignorance and poverty resulting in people becoming obese because their diet consists of too much carbohydrate and too little protein, fruit and green vegetables.

2   Lack of mobility due to degenerative diseases common in old age often as a result of poor nutrition in earlier years.

3   Familial tendencies and endocrine factors.

4   The habit of taking snacks between meals.

5   Life-long habit of overeating, possibly as a consequence of boredom and a refuge from unhappiness.

Some people in middle age regard being overweight at this period in their lives as a sign of good health!

Some of the following complications may occur in the elderly who have become obese since middle age:

1   Diabetes. Mature onset diabetes often occurs as a result of the pancreas being unable to cope with the increased carbohydrate intake in the body.

2   Fatty generation of the heart muscle, with resulting angina and hypertension.

3   Heart failure with dependent oedema and leg ulceration.

4   Chronic bronchitis and emphysema.

5   Degenerative arthritis of the weight-bearing joints.

6   Complications are more likely to develop following surgery.

7   Successful rehabilitation is far more difficult to achieve following fractured femur or cerebrovascular accident.

8   If confined to bed, the patient is far more likely to develop a

pressure sore, deep vein thrombosis or pulmonary embolism. These elderly cause extra stress to their families if they become ill and require nursing.

Prevention and treatment

1   Education in earlier years can prevent obesity occurring, with people being encouraged to eat a good staple diet with well balanced nutrients.

2   In consultation with the dietitian, the patient may be given a 4200 kJ diet and supplements of iron, calcium and vitamins. See Table 2 at end of chapter.

3   Patient and relatives shoul co-operate fully—biscuits, cakes and sweets should be discouraged.

4   A regular weight record should be kept to ensure weight is being lost and to encourage the patient.

5   When some weight has been lost, a normal diet should be encouraged.

Education in healthy eating can be given by the health visitor or at day centres and hospitals. Patients in hospital should also receive help from the dietitian.

Constipation

Constipation is a common complaint among the general population as well as the elderly. Poor diet is a common cause of constipation and education in this field can improve the situation. The following points should be observed:

1   Adequate fluids should be taken— 1 to 1½ litres daily. Fear of incontinence often prevents this and much encouragement should be given in this sphere.

2   Diet should contain fibre and cellulose. These are needed to ensure good bowel movement by maintaining the muscle tone and increasing bulk. The elderly should be encouraged to use wholemeal flour and bread as opposed to white flour and bread.

EATING IN INSTITUTIONS

For many of those living in homes and hospitals mealtimes are one of the highlights of the day, and so it is important that the staff do everything possible to make these pleasant, social occasions. The following points should be remembered:

1   Meals should be small and well presented, and where

possible the patient should be provided with what he feels he can eat.

2   The food should be hot.

3   Meals should be served in a congenial atmosphere and a social occasion made of them. Where possible a choice should be available and patients/residents should help themselves.

4   Where possible the tables should be attractively laid with cloths and flowers should be displayed. Table napkins should be used.

5   Some may not be able to eat solid food because they are edentulous, or have ill fitting false teeth, or have difficulty swallowing. These patients may benefit from having their diet liquidized or puréed.

6   For those only able to take liquid foods, there are several varieties now on the market which contain all the nutrients required hidden in an enticing flavour.

7   It is important that the handicapped patient be placed in the most comfortable position for meals, so that he can enjoy them and wherever possible feed himself. Only when really necessary should the patient be fed as this is a very degrading process. Where feeding is necessary, the nurse should be seated, give the patient her full attention, and appear unhurried.

8   Those who are disabled or need an aid should be assessed by the occupational therapist and the most suitable implements provided, e.g. non-slip mats, plate bunkers, special cutlery.

9   Those requiring special diets should be seen by the dietitian.

10   For those living permanently in institutions a variety in the diet is always welcome. Homemade cakes, strawberries, wine and cheese or fish and chips (out of a newspaper!) are generally appreciated.

11   Moderate alcohol should be encouraged—beer, and a glass of wine or sherry are often much appreciated and act as appetizers.

INTRAGASTRIC FEEDING

The unconscious patient must be fed by an intragastric tube, a suitable diet having been devised. Feeds are generally given 2-hourly during the day and less frequently at night. A fluid intake of 2 litres should be adequate unless there are contra-indications requiring more or less fluid. The energy value is worked out according to the patient's needs, and the feeds prepared by the dietitian. In some cases a fine-bore tube can be passed and a proprietary feed given.

The tube is usually passed and left in situ, being changed 2 or 3 times a week. The patient will be placed in the recumbent position with the head raised and tilted forward. Whether the patient is conscious or not a clear explanation will be given by the nurse before starting the procedure. The tube is passed through the nostril to the stomach, and if the patient is co-operative he can be asked to swallow at the appropriate time. If the tube should enter either bronchus, the patient will immediately cough or become cyanosed and the tube must be withdrawn at once. When the tube is in place the nurse must check with a registered nurse that it is in fact in the correct position. This can be done by aspirating part of the stomach content and testing it for acidity, or placing a funnel on the end of the tube and inverting it in some water. If the tube is in the bronchus bubbles will be seen and the water will rise and fall in the funnel on inspiration and expiration. When it is clear that the tube is correctly placed in the stomach, the tube is secured in position with some adhesive tape and a spigot placed in the end.

Before giving a feed, the patient will be turned on his side so that if he vomits, he will not inhale his vomit. He should always be turned before, not after, the feed, as turning on a full stomach may cause the patient to vomit. The tube should be checked before every feed, as it is very easy for it to enter the trachea without causing any distress to the patient. The feed should be given at a temperature of 37°C (98.5°F) and slowly so as not to overload the stomach.

INTRAVENOUS FEEDING

On admission to hospital, the elderly patient is often dehydrated and requires rehydration before treatment for the specific disease can begin. It is often far more beneficial to the patient to give intravenous fluids for 24–48 hours than to struggle with oral fluids for the reluctant drinker. The intravenous fluids will be prescribed by the doctor and will also correct the electrolyte imbalance which may have occurred. Intravenous feeding may be necessary for some time for those patients who cannot tolerate food by mouth or nasogastric tube. This is an expensive form of feeding which is also very irritable to the vein and is only used when no other form of feeding is possible.

Carbohydrate is given as fructose or glucose and the most common is 30% sorbitol, supplying 5000 kJ per litre. Fat emulsion is derived from cotton seed oil and soya bean oil. One litre of 10% fat emulsion, with the addition of 5% sorbitol to render it isotonic, will provide 7500 kJ.

Protein is provided in the form of amino acids. These are usually combined in one preparation which combines amino acids and fructose and provides 3400 kJ/litre.

In many cases it may be necessary to keep an accurate fluid balance chart. Fluid intake and output should be measured and charted. The dietary regimen will be recorded in the care plan.

Thus it can be seen that both over- and undernourishment are encountered when treating the elderly. Undernourishment is usually correctable and the elderly will respond well to treatment. However, the adverse effects of overnourishment are often more long-standing and difficult to treat. Education needs to take place from school years to encourage and stimulate people to follow a nutritious diet.

Further reading

Beck, M.E. (1980) *Nutrition and Dietetics for Nurses*, 6th edition. Edinburgh: Churchill Livingstone.

Davies, L. (1981) *Three Score Years and Then? A Study of the Nutrition and Well-being of Elderly People at Home*. London: Heinemann Medical.

Nursing—the Add-on Journal of Clinical Nursing. Aug./Sept. 1982—Nutrition.

Shackleton, A.D. & Poleman, C.L. (1979) *Practical Nurse Nutrition Education*. Philadelphia: W.B. Saunders.

Table 2. Weight-reducing programme (allowing an intake of approximately 4200 kJ)

Daily allowance	½ pt (500 ml) milk ½ oz (14 g) butter *or* margarine 3 oz (85 g) bread
Breakfast	Fresh grapefruit *or* small orange *or* 4 oz (120 ml) unsweetened fruit juice (small glass) 1 egg, boiled or poached *or* 1 oz (28 g) grilled bacon (1 rasher) Tomato *or* mushroom, as liked 1 oz (28 g) bread Scraping of butter (*or* margarine) from allowance Tea *or* coffee, with milk from allowance
Mid-morning	Tea *or* coffee, with milk from allowance *or* Bovril *or* Oxo *or* Marmite
Dinner at mid-day or evening	3 oz (84 g) lean meat with unthickened gravy *or* 5 oz (140 g) fish Green vegetables, as liked Root vegetables (e.g. carrot, beetroot) 1 tablespoon 1 portion fresh or stewed fruit
Mid-afternoon	1 oz (28 g) bread Scraping of butter (*or* margarine) from allowance Salad vegetable *or* Marmite Tea with milk from allowance
Supper or lunch	3 oz (84 g) lean meat with unthickened gravy *or* 5 oz (140 g) fish *or* 1½ oz (42 g) cheese *or* 2 eggs Green vegetables *or* salad, as liked 1 oz (28 g) bread Scraping of butter (*or* margarine) from allowance 1 portion fresh or stewed fruit
Bedtime	Tea *or* coffee, with milk from allowance *or* Bovril *or* Oxo *or* Marmite

9
Rehabilitation

Rehabilitation is very much an exercise in team work, and the successful outcome of the patient's treatment depends upon the ability of the members of the team to work well together. The leader of the team must obviously be the physician in charge, and the work is shared amongst the nursing staff, occupational therapists, physiotherapists, speech therapists and social workers. In some units rehabilitation aides may also be used. These are people trained specifically in rehabilitation who work within the departments and the wards. Important members of the team also are the porters and ambulance drivers who transport the patients and play a big part in making their visit enjoyable, and the chiropodist, because unless the patient's feet are well cared for, he is unable even to attempt to walk. For many patients the clergy too may have an important role to play in their care at this stage. In order to work more closely with these people the nurse must understand the principles of the therapists' work, but first of all, we shall consider the role of the nurse herself.

The nurse

In many ways the nurse has the most important role in the rehabilitation team as she is with the patient 24 hours per day and thus has to continue the work of the other specialists in the team. She is responsible for all the activities of daily living such as washing, dressing and eating, and she will help the patient to identify his particular problems and solve them where possible with the help of the specialists.

It is the nurse's responsibility to see that the ground which the patient has gained in a short period of treatment with one of the rehabilitation specialists, i.e. the physiotherapist or occupational therapist, is extended during the rest of the patient's day and at the weekend. Most nurses now receive some training from the physiotherapist in the basic techniques of transferring a patient from bed to chair, and from chair to commode. They learn the correct way to help a patient up from a chair on to a walking-aid, and the importance of ensuring that he has got his balance before he moves off (Figs. 20 and 21). The nurse can learn from the physiotherapist the way to prevent a frozen shoulder in a hemiplegic patient, simply by elevating the patient's weak arm whenever she attends to him for any reason.

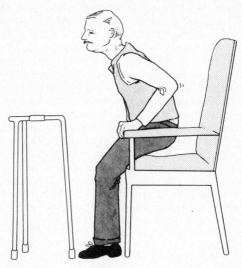

Figure 20. Correct way for an elderly patient to rise from a chair.

Similarly with dressing, the detailed assessment of a patient with a dressing disability takes a very long time and is primarily work for the occupational therapist. But as the patient improves the work can be taken over by the nurse. She can assist him by seeing that his clothes are in proper order. She must not retard his progress by taking over the whole job herself in order to save time unless he is completely helpless.

The occupational therapist

The occupational therapist assesses the functional disability of

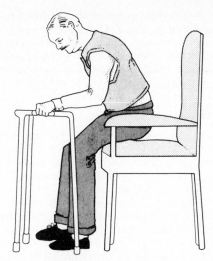

Figure 21. Incorrect way for an elderly patient to rise from a chair.

the patient in relation to the activities of daily living, watching the patient dressing, getting in and out of bed, off the lavatory, in and out of the bath, cooking and washing up. She will advise and give assistance where necessary, and will teach the patient how best to cope with his disability. She will also teach the relatives how they can best manage the patient's problems when the time comes for him to go home, and they may come and spend a day in the occupational therapy department. None of this can be done unless the occupational therapist has knowledge of the patient's home conditions. She may visit the home to assess the situation and to determine whether there is need for any alterations or improvements. She will note whether the patient has a chair, bed and lavatory at the right height and, where there are stairs, whether it will be possible for the patient to get up and down them.

The occupational therapist also provides and supervises exercises for specific disabilities. For instance, various forms of basket-making provide exercises for the joints of the hands and fingers. Weaving and loom work teach co-ordination of hands and eyes and provide some work for the arms to do. Working on large looms involves both arms and legs.

The therapist will want to know what goal the patient is aiming for, so this must be clearly defined by the whole team, and if necessary a time limit must be set so that everyone is aware of the objective. Group activities will also be included in her work, and these enable the patient to communicate with others and give a sense of purpose and belonging.

The physiotherapist

Regular physiotherapy is not only valuable but indeed essential treatment in the majority of diseases encountered on the geriatric ward, e.g. patients suffering from cerebrovascular accident with resulting hemiplegia, parkinsonism, varicose ulcers, arthritis, fracture and amputation.

The physiotherapist must first assess the patient's condition and teach him how to become mobile again, providing him with a suitable aid as necessary. Once he has learned to walk again, he can quickly regain much more independence. Secondly, the physiotherapist is concerned with maintenance of function in those patients with a long-standing disability such as osteoarthrosis, who have developed another condition such as diabetes or heart failure, which may require a period of investigation and even immobilization in hospital. This may result in weakness or contractures and loss of former mobility. Thirdly, the physiotherapist may also give specific exercises for various disabilities and disuse of muscles and joints. She may be required to give infra-red heat and ultraviolet light for specific lesions.

Her work is closely aligned to that of the occupational therapist, but the nursing staff must also work with her as they must carry on the patient's treatment in the absence of the physiotherapist. All members of the nursing staff must be aware of the patient's capabilities, and what aids and how many people are required to help the patient walk or transfer from bed to chair. There should be some indication in writing of all this (e.g. the care plan), which should be placed in the ward where everyone can refer to it, thus avoiding confusion.

The speech therapist

The speech therapist concentrates on the patient with speech defects, generally following cerebrovascular accident or where there is a cerebral lesion. She will work with the patients individually and in groups to help them overcome their disabilities and learn to communicate again with those around them.

When the speech therapist is working on the wards the nurse must allow her a quiet corner so that the patient is not distracted by noise and activity around her, and can concentrate fully on the training.

The social worker

The social worker has an important function in the team while the patient is being rehabilitated. She must co-operate with all the staff and attend to the patient's financial and home commitments, and allay any fears concerning these that may arise. She liaises between staff and relatives to see that suitable clothes and shoes are available for the patient. She will also assist in the patient's future. She will help organize the home if necessary to see that all is ready for the patient's return and liaise with the social services department of the local authority if any alterations need to be made. If the patient is unable to return home and suitable accommodation must be found, application may have to be made to the local authority for residential accommodation. In this case the patient must be fitted into a suitable home where the staff can meet the patient's needs, and the patient will find congenial company, so that both he and his relatives are happy in the arrangement.

General principles of rehabilitation

First, rehabilitation must be considered in the wider aspects of caring for the elderly, so that the aims and objects of the rehabilitation team can be seen as a whole. The problems of the elderly start to exert an influence on health with the passing of years—resistance to disease is diminished, as is the ability to adapt to physical and environmental change. Recovery is slower with acute problems complicated by the residual effects of previous diseases. Physiological function, perhaps a truer guide to age rather than actual years, diminishes; social support becomes less available and less reliant than to the younger patient. Maintenance of the elderly in their own homes concerns the use of both human and material resources which in some cases may involve more than one authority, and many different departments, and lead to the giving of perhaps 26 different types of services. This is a complicated and often unco-ordinated system, confusing to the patient and frustrating to the rehabilitation team.

Needs of the elderly
The needs of the elderly can be discussed under four main headings.
1 Health—to be active and comfortable.
2 Social—to be adequately supported in the community.
3 Occupational—to have a continuing role in society.
4 Spiritual—to be able to continue to develop as an individual.

None of these needs can be neglected, and whilst geriatric medicine concentrates on the first—health—the geriatrician will, through statutory and voluntary organizations, co-ordinate the others.

Assessing the needs
The assessment and recording of the needs of the elderly patient is a multidisciplinary task initiated by the geriatrician, usually at a case conference. A useful method of recording and updating data is illustrated in Fig. 22.

1 *Health:*
   a Physical—diagnosis (often multiple) and treatment.
      Prognosis—chance of cure or palliation, motivation of patient.
      Degree of disability—urinary control, bowel function, hearing, sight, teeth, feet and nails, speech.
      Effects of medication.
      Mental—Acute brain failure
              Chronic brain failure.

2 *Social:*
   Housing—heating and lighting.
   Aids and adaptations.
   Meals.
   Social work and community support.
   Day centre or day hospital.

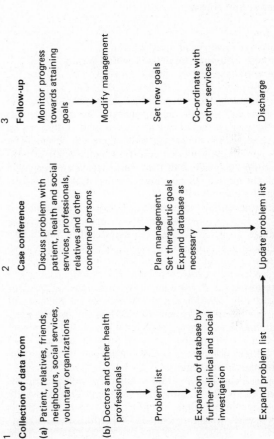

1

Collection of data from

(a) Patient, relatives, friends, neighbours, social services, voluntary organizations

(b) Doctors and other health professionals

Problem list

Expansion of database by further clinical and social investigation

Expand problem list → Update problem list

2

Case conference

Discuss problem with patient, health and social services, professionals, relatives and other concerned persons

Plan management
Set therapeutic goals
Expand database as necessary

3

Follow-up

Monitor progress towards attaining goals

Modify management

Set new goals

Co-ordinate with other services

Discharge

Figure 22. Assessing the needs of the elderly patient.

3 *Financial:*
  a Income—pensions (state and occupational), supplementary benefit, statutory allowances.
  b Capital—value of house, bank accounts, building society shares, unit trusts.

4 *Spiritual:*
Capacity to develop as an individual.
Future role within the family and within society.
Leisure activities.

Having assessed these aspects the team should then set realistic goals and plan the management of the patient accordingly. These goals should not be set too high as this can be disheartening, both to the patient and to the teams. It should be remembered too that needs are perceived by the observers and may not always coincide with the 'wants' which are perceived by the patient himself. In carrying out an accurate assessment, this should be discovered!

The team should also concentrate on capability and not on disability. It may in some cases be more appropriate to talk of 'disadvantage' as this implies less permanence than 'disability'. We are all disadvantaged at some stage in our life, some more so than others! Physically the team needs to concentrate on maintaining and improving the muscle power of the patient and actively restoring and developing muscle functions. The patient has to regard rehabilitation as a full-time job and all members of the team, including the patient, should understand the goal. The requirements of a successful rehabilitation unit are plenty of space and a well trained staff, and success depends upon maximal patient co-operation with the patient becoming the central member of the team.

After assessment and a period of intensive rehabilitation it may be necessary for an aid to be supplied. This is usually prescribed by the consultant if he decides that the patient is unable to manage without such help. When this is so, acceptance of the aid depends upon an early decision to use it, its efficiency and the understanding, motivation and co-operation of the patient in learning to use it.

Appliances

An appliance is a device made to fit the patient in order to correct a deformity or increase a function, e.g. corsets, calipers, surgical footwear and splints.

Corsets are often supplied in cases of osteoporosis and osteoarthrosis of the spine, giving good support, helping the patient when walking, and possibly relieving pain when sitting.

Calipers are sometimes required by patients following a cerebrovascular accident and in cases of footdrop and peroneal weakness which may occur after surgery or prolonged bed rest. These are usually only prescribed after a period of intensive rehabilitation, as considerable functional improvement may occur with exercise.

Surgical footwear, consisting of both boots and shoes, is generally supplied to those with ankle weakness due to hemiplegia, severe osteoarthrosis, rheumatoid arthritis and foot deformities.

Splints may be required for the arthritic or hemiplegic patient to ensure good position during periods of bed rest and enforced rest. In the case of the patient with rheumatoid arthritis, it may be necessary to rest the joint concerned for some time until the inflammation subsides. Occasionally when weakness of the wrist occurs, it may be necessary to use a splint for stabilization to help the patient to feed independently.

Personal aids consist of small items to assist functional ability, e.g. pick up sticks, bath aids, toilet aids, eating aids, household gadgets and adapted clothing. Most of these are given only after considerable assessment and active exercises as they can result in ultimate lessening of function, and if this function can be maintained for a little longer, it is ultimately to the patient's advantage.

Washing and bathing

Many patients can manage to wash partially without assistance, but the nurse may well need to give help to wash feet, backs and perineal area. For many of the elderly, baths are dangerous and should not be attempted alone at home without help from the community nurse or a relative. So often the patient finds he can get into the bath quite easily, but cannot get out alone. A shower is a suitable form of toilet for the elderly, although often not appreciated by the older generation.

Bath aids consist of various seats that enable the patient to get in and out without too much difficulty, and to lower themselves into the bath slowly. There are also various rails which can be fixed by the local authority to enable safer entry and exit to the bath.

Lavatory aids consist of a variety of rails and seat raises which can easily be fixed, as most patients find difficulty in rising from the modern, rather low lavatory.

Clothing

Adapted clothing is often very necessary and much is now readily available. Dresses with slits down the side or back and a fly-away panel are on the market, and are usually made of easily washable material needing no ironing. They are much easier to manage than pulling up a tight skirt or trying to sit elegantly in such a skirt. Similarly, trousers are made in Terylene, which is easy to wash, and have a Velcro fastening.

Shoes may prove a problem as leather may become stiff and hard due to incontinence of urine. However, there are various synthetic lace-up shoes available which are also washable and wear reasonably well. Various other garments may be adapted by the occupational therapists to various patients' individual needs, as no two people have precisely the same disabilities and difficulties.

Equipment

This consists of larger mechanical aids, hoists, special beds, adapted kitchen equipment, special chairs and remote control equipment such as the Possum (Patient-Operated Selector Mechanism) which can control doors, television, radio, tape recorder, typewriter, etc. All this is very expensive equipment, and responsibility for its supply rests with the consultant and the social services department of the local authority. The discretionary powers of local authorities are very wide-ranging, from provision of personal aids to architectural reconstruction of the patient's home, building ramps, widening doors and installing hoists. Financial arrangements vary considerably from authority to authority as does the ease with which aids are available.

The practical application of the principles of good rehabilitation can usefully be illustrated by studying a case history.

Mrs B., aged 82, was admitted from home having collapsed that morning. She was conscious but drowsy and had evidence of a right hemiparesis, having a little movement in her arm and leg. That evening she was seen by the physiotherapist and some active and passive movements were carried out on the patient's arms and legs. While in bed the affected limbs were kept in a good position, and a bed cradle was placed in the bed to relieve pressure on the feet and heels and to enable exercises to be carried out with ease.

During the next 2 days Mrs B. appeared to be making good progress and was able to sit in a chair for short periods. She had only minimal weakness in her leg and her balance was good, and the nurses were able to teach her the correct way to transfer from bed to chair. From the beginning she always wore a good pair of lace-up shoes which her daughter had brought in for her. There appeared to be very little movement in her arm and the physiotherapist taught her various exercises which she could do while sitting in a chair. A suitable chair (Fig. 23) was provided with a straight back and arms, so that the patient could up without too much difficulty. (The ward needs to have a variety of geriatric chairs, as different chairs suit different patients; some require a higher chair than others and some appreciate a foot rest, while the more active no longer have need of this. To ensure maximum independence also the bed needs to be of a suitable height, so that the patient is able to get in and out unaided if possible.)

When Mrs B. began to walk, she needed the support of two members of staff, usually the physiotherapist and a nurse, but the staff felt that it was essential that she became independent as soon as possible, and this was done by providing her with a quadriped which she soon learnt to use, firstly with an aide and then alone.

Walking is dependent on the strength and endurance of the patient. Difficulty in walking may occur in various diseases. The hemiplegic patient may experience difficulties due to interference of balance, muscle weakness and spasticity. Balance may be disturbed as a result of lesions of the cerebellar system or visual impairment. There may be weakness of the muscles of the trunk, abdomen, hip, knee or foot, and this may have an effect on walking.

Some patients do not progress well with walking and may be considered for a wheelchair after all other efforts to get the patient mobile have failed. Sometimes an ordinary small wheelchair may be sufficient for a relative to push the patient longer distances. Self-propelled wheelchairs are available with aid wheels on both or either side depending upon the handicap. The chairs have to be carefully fitted according to the patient's measurements and disability. For those with a severe disability an electric wheelchair may be necessary with

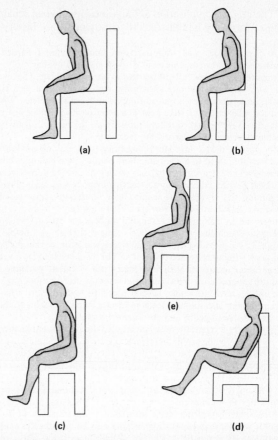

Figure 23. Suitable and unsuitable chairs. Seat (a) too broad, (b) too narrow, (c) too high, (d) too low. (e) A good fit.

convenient hand controls. When a wheelchair is considered, the home must also be examined to ensure that this is practicable there, and to see whether any alterations need to be made to accommodate the chair.

However, Mrs B. managed well with her quadriped; all the nursing staff knew that she could use this aid and that she was considered safe to walk alone. While Mrs B. was learning to walk, she was also learning to use the lavatory unaided, to feed and dress herself. The nurse, physiotherapist and occupational therapist all worked together and Mrs B. attended the occupational therapy department two or three mornings a week to pursue her activities. Mrs B. was encouraged to be dressed in her own clothes early on during her stay, as this has a remarkable effect on the patient's morale. The daughter was advised to bring in dresses which had easy access, as Mrs B. still had little movement in her right arm, making dressing a difficult procedure.

Mrs B. did have some problems when eating and drinking as she had to manage this left-handed. She was never encouraged to be fed, as this can be very degrading and frustrating for the patient. She found it much easier to manage when sitting in a chair, and was therefore always up for supper and breakfast. Sometimes the diet can be adapted to the benefit of the patient and help may be obtained from the dietitian and catering officer, e.g. salads are difficult to manage unless shredded, soups are easier to manage if they are thicker and can be drunk from a cup rather than from a bowl. Mrs B. was provided with a Nelson knife which incorporated a cutting device and a fork. The staff always ensured that her plate was placed on a non-slip mat, so she did not have to worry about it sliding about the table, and she always had a plate bunker or Manoy bowl, so that she did not have to chase the food round the plate thus allowing it to become unnecessarily cold.

Speech

The speech therapist will treat patients with speech difficulties which occur mainly in the following groups of patients: those with Parkinson's disease and parkinsonism, motor neuron disease, cerebral lesions and following cerebrovascular accidents. She will treat those with disturbances of language, articulation, voice and swallowing. Before beginning treatment she must assess the degree of disability and during the detailed assessment many problems, not always so obvious to the nurse, will be highlighted. The assessment will include the ability to understand, express speech, articulate words, and move tongue and lips. Some of the following disabilities may be present.

Dysarthria is a neuromuscular problem which affects the power of speech either partially or completely. It results in slurred, weakly articulated sounds and although the meaning of the words is quite clear, the production is not.

Dysphasia is the partial loss of the ability to speak and understand speech and *aphasia* is the complete loss of this ability. *Motor aphasia* occurs when the patient fails to put his thoughts into recognizable words, but can understand all that is said to him. *Sensory aphasia* occurs when the patient cannot understand the written or spoken word and then there is great difficulty in any form of communication. These patients should not be treated as though they had dementia, but need much patience, understanding and skill. Some of them are very good at understanding gestures and following clues. They tend to become cut off from the surrounding world, often suffering frustration and depression.

Apraxia is the inability to fit movements together to carry out a useful activity and *agnosia* the inability to identify the purpose of objects and sounds. Both are sometimes first diagnosed by the speech therapist during her assessment.

Dysphonia is a reduction in volume of speech due to disorders of the respiratory or laryngeal muscles. It results in the voice becoming very quiet or hoarse.

All the treatment required has to be tailor-made for the patient by the speech therapist and nurses must be aware of the lines of treatment so that they can continue to help the patients in the ward during their everyday duties of feeding, dressing and bathing them. It is a very individual form of treatment and therefore very time-consuming.

Group therapy for the speech handicapped should be encouraged as this method is of proved psychological as well as clinical benefit.

Rehabilitation of the elderly amputee

This is commonly undertaken these days in the geriatric unit and specialized care before and after surgery will ensure good results.

Preoperatively the patient's physical condition will be assessed, especially his cardiovascular and respiratory systems. The patient must also receive good psychological preparation, a thorough explanation being given to both the patient and the relatives. It may often help if the patient can be visited by a previous amputee who is now home and independent. However, on no account should false hopes be raised. The loss of part of a limb following amputation can be compared to loss of a close member of the family and the period of readjustment may take several months. The reaction of the staff and family to the patient before and following amputation can have a great influence on the period of rehabilitation.

The patient may have to be transferred to a surgical ward for the actual operation and the first few postoperative days. Pain should be relieved immediately postoperatively and regularly thereafter. The nursing staff should be alert to the fact that the patient may be a little confused for the first 24–48 hours after operation.

The stump should be well bandaged as this helps to keep a good shape, produce less pain and prevent oedema. The site of the amputation depends on the cause of the operation and the blood supply to the limb. It is usually easiest to rehabilitate those who have a through-knee amputation. If infection is already present, it may be necessary to perform delayed suturing. The majority of these patients are diabetic and therefore healing is slower and the risk of infection may be greater. Infection can lead to oedema, haematoma and osteomyelitis. It is also important for future limb fitting that there is a viable stump flap. Exercises should be given at once after operation, with extension of the limb and prone-lying to prevent flexion. Arm muscles may be improved by the use of a monkey chain and pole.

The patient should be up in a chair as soon as possible and in a wheelchair within a week of surgery. He should be hopping with a walking-frame fairly quickly. Provided the stump heals without delay, the patient may visit the limb-fitting centre for the first fitting 2 weeks after surgery and have the limb 2 weeks after that. Depending upon the centre, the patient may have a leg immediately, or may first have a pylon and then a leg. Depending also on the patient's capabilities, the physician in charge of the case may feel that he is not fit to graduate from pylon to leg and that the change is not beneficial to the patient.

Mental rehabilitation

It has already been emphasized that mental activities and attitudes are as important as physical exercise and training. If the elderly patient is depressed and can see no future in living with his disability, no amount of physical activity will achieve any good result. In an active, optimistic atmosphere much can be achieved with the willing co-operation of the patient. In the initial stages this can be hard to attain and help may be sought from the social worker and hospital chaplain. The latter has a part to play as a listener and advisor liaising, in some cases, between patient and staff.

Group therapy in the rehabilitation unit too instils the will to improve and also prepares the patient to accept his degree of disability or disadvantage. A short period during the afternoon may be devoted to group therapy and must be carefully organized by the nursing staff, occupational therapists, well supervised voluntary workers or a youth club. Communal activities such as card games, dominoes, bingo, music and movement, frieze work or even folding plastic bags may be enjoyed, as may occasionally viewing a few carefully selected slides. In the female ward hairdressing sessions and manicures may be appreciated too.

However, perhaps the best therapy is the happy home life to which the patient is anxious to return. This may be maintained in hospital if visiting is unrestricted and the nursing staff encourage the relatives to visit whenever possible and to help as much as they like and feel able. The help, however, must be constant and not overprotective, as this is sometimes the cause of the patient's being in hospital initially. The unit must not become isolated and outside visits should be arranged whenever practical and possible.

Further reading

Dardier, E.M. (1980) *The Early Stroke Patient—Positioning and Movement.* London: Baillière Tindall.

Disabled Living Foundation (1975) *Kitchen Sense.* London: Heinemann Medical.

Eaton, G.V. (1975) *A Stroke in the Family.* New York: Wildwood House.

Humm, W. (1977) *Rehabilitation of the Lower Limb Amputee: For Nurses and Therapists.* London: Baillière Tindall.

Johnson, M. (1976) *The Stroke Patient: Principles of Rehabilitation.* Edinburgh: Churchill Livingstone.

Mattingley, S. (1977) *Rehabilitation Today.* London: Update.

Stewart, M.C. (1971) *My Brother's Keeper*, 2nd edition. London: Health Horizon.

10
Mental Disorders and Mental Illness

The incidence of disease and disability rises with age, and especially sharply over the age of 75. The most common diseases affect sight, hearing, maintenance of continence, and the joints. However, one in seven people over the age of 75 suffer from some degree of mental disorder, particularly dementia and depression (*Growing Older*, 1981). Elderly people over the age of 65 form the largest single group of in-patients under the care of the psychiatric hospital service, most of these suffering from mental infirmity directly connected with the problems of ageing, and it is estimated that approximately two thirds of the patients in psychiatric hospitals will soon be over the age of 65.

Many natural changes occur in the brain during the course of growing old and these include failure of memory, so that incidents which happened many years ago are much clearer than those that occurred quite recently. The elderly person may also experience difficulty with the interpretation of stimuli; thus bowel and bladder control may become impaired and reactions to taste, smell and pain may be dulled. As we grow older, we find it harder to adapt to new situations, so a change of environment and admission to hospital may have an adverse effect on the elderly, which some take longer to overcome than others. There may also be instability of mental function and a weakening of emotional control whereby the patient may more easily be reduced to tears.

So often when caring for the elderly any evidence of confusion or disorientation is quickly and incorrectly referred to as 'senile dementia' and no further attempt is made to investigate the cause or relieve the symptoms.

Acute confusion

This occurs when the patient can no longer understand or make sense of his social and physical circumstances. It is a very common cause of admission to hospital and it is often forgotten that confusion is a symptom underlying a disease and not a disease in itself.

Causes

a) Infection   This is a very common cause of acute confusion, often accompanied by a rise in temperature. Chest and urinary tract infections are usually the most common infections responsible for confusion. They may produce few other symptoms except for a period of disorientation. Once the underlying infection has been treated or treatment has commenced, the confusion will clear.

b) Cerebral anoxia   This may be due to an acute disturbance of the blood supply to the brain following a cerebrovascular accident or to failure of the oxygen supply to the brain caused by heart failure, respiratory failure, anaemia or myocardial infarction.

c) Cerebral hypoxia   (diminished supply of oxygen to the brain)   This may exist for a very short period following surgery and can cause damage to the already somewhat precarious brain cells. It may take a patient a little while to compensate for such damage, and thus it is extremely common for a period of confusion to follow surgical intervention. When emergency surgery is performed the nurse must remember that the patient may have been rushed into hospital, into strange surroundings, seen by innumerable different people and taken to theatre all within the space of 24–48 hours, so that he will already be confused on this account.

d) Disorders of metabolism   Confusion may be caused by dehydration, renal failure, diabetes (especially if the patient becomes hypoglycaemic), myxoedema, and hypothermia. In many of these cases the confusion may progress to coma.

e) Deficiency disorders   Confusion may also occur with lack of vitamins of the B complex. Once the diagnosis has been established and replacement therapy begun, a rapid improvement will be evident in 10–14 days. The usual treatment is a course of intravenous or intramuscular Parentrovite.

f) Disorientation due to unfamiliar surroundings   This often causes confusion, especially if the elderly person is partially sighted or deaf. The patient who is used to living alone in a small house will be completely bewildered by the spaciousness of a hospital ward, the innumerable different faces and the continuous activity. Introductions and a guided tour of the ward may help.

g) Drugs   These are a common cause of acute confusion in the elderly. If the patient suddenly becomes confused after the start of a new treatment, the nurse must report the fact to the doctor and the cause must be investigated. If a new drug or drugs have been commenced this should be noted and the dosage reduced if necessary. Frequently the patient has become confused before admission to hospital, and has had large doses of drugs which have resulted in the confusional state, e.g. some tranquillizers, including the phenothiazine group of drugs, antidepressants, especially imipramine and amitriptyline, antiparkinsonian drugs, digoxin, some vasodilators, which may improve the blood supply to a specific area by 'stealing' from the rest of the body, and sedatives, particularly barbiturates. Great care should be taken at night to give sedation only when really necessary and to avoid barbiturates unless the patient has been accustomed to taking them for some time with no ill effects.

h) Full bowel or bladder   The nurse must remember that this is a common cause of acute confusion.

i) Acute confusion   may also occur in the patient with an infection superimposed on a chronic disease, resulting in a chronic shortage of oxygen supply to the brain, for instance in chronic heart disease, chronic lung disease and narrowing of the arteries by atheroma or blockage.

All these causes may result in delirium with lack of awareness of events around the patient, illusions and hallucinations which may become more marked at night. The less severe confusional state may last for some weeks even months.

Treatment
In view of the many possible causes of confusional states in the elderly, the underlying cause must be discovered before a course of treatment is initiated. When treatment is begun it may be helpful to add vitamin supplements, given by intravenous or intramuscular routes.

The nurse must bear in mind the typical picture of the old man admitted to hospital and put to bed. He suddenly has an urge to micturate and tries to get out of bed. He wanders down the ward, is immediately put back to bed, cot sides are erected and he is heavily sedated. Thus he awakens in the morning far more confused and disorientated. How much simpler it would have been for the enlightened nurse to have shown the patient the way to the lavatory, then taken him to the kitchen, made a cup of tea and had a chat before taking the old man back to bed.

The elderly population must be kept in touch with reality, given their spectacles and encouraged to read the newspaper. Wearing their own clothes, too, helps them to retain their sense of personal identity and the surroundings will appear less strange if peopled with normally dressed individuals. It is important that the nursing staff always address patients by their proper names and not by familiar terms of endearment. Bathrooms and lavatories must be clearly indicated, either with colours or with labels in large lettering, and entrance and exit signs should be marked on the doors, inside as well as outside. The nurse must be aware of the reason for any disorientation that may occur and be prepared to expect this.

The patient must be allowed to do what he likes provided this is safe, and he must not be forcibly restrained. Over-sedation must be avoided; if necessary a little promazine may be given for a few days and usually this will be sufficient.

Relatives must be warned and the reason for the confusion explained, as it may be very distressing for them to arrive and find that their elderly relative does not recognize them or appears to be unaware of his surroundings and the period of time in which he is living.

Dementia

Statistics show that dementia affects as many as 1 in 10 people over the age of 65, which means about ¾ million people, and of those in the 80+ age group, 20% can expect to suffer dementia

(Cox 1983). This is caused by pathological changes affecting the brain tissue itself, the most common types being arteriosclerotic and senile dementia. Very often these are interrelated in varying degrees.

Arteriosclerotic dementia is caused by brain cell atrophy, secondary to arteriosclerosis and a diminishing blood supply. Blood vessels become inelastic, irregular, thickened and narrowed, thus diminishing the flow of blood, and this occurs as a result of ageing alone or because of raised blood pressure and also through dietetic factors. The result is a general dementia with loss of specific brain functions such as speech, voluntary movements of the limbs or an appreciation of sensations.

Senile dementia is caused by brain cell atrophy accompanied by unique microscopic changes, the cause of which is unknown. The patient is unable to remember recent events and suffers from disorientation of time, place and person. He will have a labile (unstable) emotional state. His personal habits become neglectful and clothes become dirty and unkempt. The patient becomes incontinent of both urine and faeces and eventually dies from bronchopneumonia. The onset is gradual and irreversible, and in arteriosclerotic dementia added cerebrovascular incidents may occur with transient paralysis and features of parkinsonism. Post-mortem examination of the brain shows general shrinking with dilatation of the ventricles, widening of the sulci (the furrows or fissures of the brain) and narrowing of the gyri (convolutions of the brain).

Pre-senile dementias

These may be seen within the geriatric unit, no other suitable accommodation having been found for the patient.

Alzheimer's disease

This is a disease resulting in premature ageing, personality changes and impaired memory. Eventually the patient is mute or incoherent. The muscles become stiff and walking is difficult, although the patient may be hyperactive. Terminally the patient is confined to bed, severely demented, totally aphasic and incontinent. There is no specific treatment other than good basic nursing care, and death results from bronchopneumonia.

Pick's disease
This is similar to Alzheimer's disease, but brain cell loss is restricted to frontal and temporal lobes. The disease is more common in women.

Huntington's chorea
This is a rare disease, and is a combination of dementia and involuntary movements due to degeneration of the cells of the cortex and extrapyramidal nuclei. It is an inherited disease due to a dominant gene.

Symptoms start between the ages of 30 and 45 years. There is a change of temperament leading to a disintegration of personality, alteration of judgement and memory failure. The limb movements become jerky, irregular and clumsy. As the disease advances walking is impossible and the patient is confined to bed with swallowing impaired. Death usually occurs about 15 years from the onset of symptoms. Some relief occurs from antiparkinsonian agents and tranquillizers.

Dementia secondary to infection
With the introduction of penicillin, the treatment of syphilis was radically changed and it is now a curable disease. It can be treated even in the tertiary stage and the syphilitic conditions described below are much more rarely seen nowadays.

In *cerebrovascular syphilis* damage is limited to the tissues covering the brain, meninges and blood vessels supplying it. The membranes become thickened and the blood vessels narrowed. Symptoms resemble those of arteriosclerotic dementia. In *tabes dorsalis*, damage is limited to the posterior tracts of the spinal cord, which causes impairment of the patient's ability to recognize where his limbs are in space. This results in difficulty in walking. *General paralysis of the insane* develops many years later with mental or physical disorders. Physical disorders include disturbances of speech with slurring of the words. In 50% of the patients, the pupils no longer constrict or dilate but respond only to accommodation.

Multiple cerebrovascular accidents and hemiplegia

These occur generally in patients who are hypertensive and may have been so for some time. Progress is slow, the patient suffers from minor strokes, transient loss of consciousness, fits, falls for no obvious reason and periods of weakness or paraesthesia. There are changes of behaviour and mentality. The patient becomes restless, bad-tempered and inconsiderate and personal cleanliness deteriorates markedly. Eventually signs of dementia develop and the disease is progressive and irreversible.

Cerebral neoplasm

This causes destruction of the surrounding brain cells and irritation of the cells through pressure on them. There is obstruction of the free flow of the cerebrospinal fluid through the ventricles and around the brain. Signs are headaches, giddiness, vomiting, slow pulse and papilloedema, which is caused by obstruction to the venous return from the retina by raised intercranial pressure, causing swelling of the optic discs. Fits occur, with progressive dementia and focal neurological signs. Tumours arising in the frontal lobes are particularly likely to produce personality changes and progressive dementia.

Anaemia

Anaemia superimposed upon an already precarious, but stable, mental state may have disastrous effects. It may increase depression and confusion and aggravate the dementia. Once the cause has been discovered, and replacement therapy begun, the patient should show signs of improvement.

Functional disorders

Anxiety state
This may show itself first in the elderly patient, but has usually occurred earlier in the patient's life and is not a new manifestation. The patient is usually over-anxious about his illness (real or imagined), and subsequent treatment, and this may result in childish behaviour and even incontinence. There may be depression, loss of appetite, and preoccupation with bodily function, with the patient eventually believing that no part of the body functions as it should.

One elderly lady admitted to hospital with severe bronchopneumonia had had a mild anxiety state for some time. Recently she had lost her husband, son and brother all within the space of 6 months and this had not helped her condition. She rapidly recovered from the broncho-pneumonia, but took some time to rehabilitate and become independent again. She had a slight tremor and profuse sweating at times. Her bowels caused her considerable agitation, as they acted infrequently and only with aid. Despite the stools being very soft and the rectum being loaded, she was unable to evacuate easily. She became more and more agitated, dwelling continuously on the number of days she had been unable to pass a stool. Eventually, with gentle persuasion, introduction of a regular routine and use of mild aperients when necessary, regular bowel habits developed and the patient was able to cope with normal defecation.

Depression
This is common in the elderly, but often tends not to be diagnosed as the elderly may have a morbid outlook on life anyway. Many patients are loath to admit that they are depressed. Causes are deafness, blindness, pain, immobility, loss of taste, poverty and, perhaps most commonly, bereavement.

One must distinguish between myxoedema and depression. In myxoedema, there may be impairment of the memory confused with pre-senile dementia, and the patient may become mentally confused or even psychotic in behaviour, but there will also be other signs and symptoms of myxoedema.

Reactive or exogenous depression There are numerous reasons for this condition, especially among patients admitted to hospital. If they live alone they may be concerned as to whether they will be able to return home and manage alone again. They become depressed at the thought of having to give up their home and perhaps live in residential accommodation or a nursing home, thus losing not only their independence but also their privacy. Some may feel rejected by their relatives, life may have been difficult at home and the family may have become resentful of their elderly relative living with them. The old person may realize this and become depressed at feeling a burden. Others may worry at the thought of having to return home to relatives whom they think cannot manage, but become depressed at the thought of having to spend the rest of their lives in hospital or a home.

Endogenous depression This has usually begun in earlier

life and persists into old age. The patients partake in few activities—everything is too much effort. They dislike food and suffer from lack of concentration. They experience delusions of guilt, poverty, hypochondria and nihilism. They may feel that part of their body is dead. These people often do better if treated at home, but not if they are suicidal or if the home environment is unsuitable.

There is a high rate of suicides in the elderly, especially amongst men, many of whom suffer from the endogenous type of depression. Contributory factors include loneliness, bereavement and physical illness. Ill-planned retirement may have some link with the higher rate among men. All threats should be taken seriously and many may need a period of hospitalization.

Signs of depression:

a   Agitation and restlessness with wandering at night.
b   Aimless wandering during the day.
c   Loss of appetite resulting in nutritional deficiencies and malnutrition.
d   Constipation.
e   Loss of interest in self and surroundings with some confusion.
f   Neglect of home and person.
g   Failure to respond to approaches or to answer questions.

Treatment   Before treating depression the doctor and nurse must first look to the cause and if possible remove or try to alleviate the problem. In the event of retirement and boredom being the cause for depression, some form of occupation in the voluntary sector may be found. Of course, pre-retirement courses are designed to help prevent this type of depression. Social workers have an active part to play here in helping to find an answer to some of the problems which result in depression. For those admitted to hospital much too will depend on the nursing staff of the ward and the atmosphere within the ward. The degree of social contact and the policy of the ward towards social activities is also important, and all need to work together to create an optimistic atmosphere where patients feel able to share their burdens and search for relief. Treatment with psychotropic drugs may be necessary or even a course of electroconvulsive therapy.

Bereavement syndrome

Severe depression may occur in the elderly who have lost a close friend or relative on whom they are dependent, particularly a spouse. It usually occurs in those who already have a tendency to depression, but generally clears with help from social workers, clergy, therapists and nurses when the patient is in hospital. However, it should be remembered that it is normal to grieve and that normal bereavement passes through several stages over a period of several weeks or months. Help and counselling may be offered by the health visitor and the general practitioner, and in many areas voluntary workers are trained especially for this situation.

Mrs B. was admitted from home having lost her husband 6 weeks previously. She was a pleasant lady who had had a history of ischaemic heart disease for several years, and mild depression at times. On the death of her husband she became acutely depressed and was now quite unable to cope alone. Initially on admission to the ward, she was quite cheerful and able, but gradually reverted to her original state of acute depression. She was visited by a psychiatrist and treatment with antidepressant drugs was commenced. Improvement became quite marked and soon she was considered fit to return home. At the mention of this she deteriorated rapidly. As she had been well able to cope at home prior to her husband's death it was decided to send her home to see how she would manage, having given her maximum support and having alerted the social services and the psychiatrist. Unfortunately the patient declined rapidly at home, and was admitted to a psychiatric hospital for another period of treatment.

Paraphrenia

This is a form of schizophrenia occurring in the elderly, especially spinsters living alone and rather isolated. They have feelings of being spied upon, and that their neighbours may be transmitting harmful rays to them. There are known cases of houses being boarded up with newspapers against this evil, so that the rays are not able to get through. Such patients are generally difficult to control.

Mania and hypomania

Patients suffering from mania or hypomania are cheerful and confident. They are supremely fit and able, and become restless and noisy if not treated. Whilst in their manic state, food and drink may be omitted and they may feel they are being poisoned. They may become more preoccupied with the cause of the manic state. Eventually if no treatment is given, they become exhausted, suffering from dehydration and malnutrition. They may be treated with parenteral tranquillizers such as haloperidol.

Management

The majority of elderly people suffering from mental disorders are best cared for in their own homes for as long as possible. It is especially essential that the demented patient be maintained in a familiar environment for as long as possible. It is also essential that such patients are given as much support as possible from community services:

a   The community psychiatric nursing services may be able to visit and offer support in conjunction with the community nursing services.
b   Home helps and meals-on-wheels will offer help with daily living activities.
c   Laundry services may be essential, especially where the elderly person is incontinent.
d   Night sitters may be necessary when nocturnal restlessness and wandering are a problem.
e   Voluntary visitors may be a great help and support.

Many of the elderly mentally infirm live with their relatives and they too will need much help and support. Caring for such people can be extremely exhausting and demoralizing and much understanding needs to be given. Watching an elderly spouse or parent become more confused and demented can be the cause of much grief and sadness.

The routine at home should be constant, so that the patient's day has a familiar pattern. The home should be undisturbed, so that furniture and familiar objects are easily recognized. For as long as possible the patient should be encouraged to be independent, to carry out simple chores and pursue old hobbies. So often relatives find it quicker and easier to help the patient with activities of daily living as these may become very slow and laborious.

Day care

Day care is not often available for the elderly mentally infirm but most psychiatric units have day hospital facilities for these people. It is often a key factor in maintaining the elderly person at home and gives the relative a well earned break. Firm friendships may be formed and the familiar routine and faces may not be too disruptive, once the initial re-organization of routines has taken place.

The day should be well planned with a friendly greeting on arrival and time over coffee to chat to the staff. Physical and mental stimulation must be included, familiar songs may be sung, and even dancing may be enjoyed. Personal care should be given much attention. Feeding may require assistance and assessment. Daily baths may be given and hairdressing, make-up and manicure all provide a boost to the patient's morale. Chiropody may be provided also, and the patient will be able to attend the physiotherapy department if necessary. A doctor will be in attendance so that medical needs may be assessed, as well as the condition of ears, eyes, feet, bladder and bowels.

Drugs

Drugs may be required to help improve the brain metabolism which has been damaged by lack of oxygen. These should be commenced very early, when deterioration is first noted. Tranquillizers, sedatives and antidepressants should all be used with extreme caution and any side-effects noted and resolved as soon as possible.

Care in hospital

Nursing management of the elderly mentally infirm is never easy. If hospital admission is necessary, 5% of these patients may go into general beds as they have some underlying physical disease. Their care is left very much to the nursing staff and an enlightened outlook is much needed if any degree of success is to be achieved.

These people are especially sensitive to disapproval or affection, so non-verbal communication is of great importance, and the formation and sustaining of a relationship with these patients is essential. Often when verbal communication seems impossible—to the patient's distress and the nurse's frustration—the effect of facial signals may well be heightened. This means that the nurse must plan and control the pitch, tone and volume of her voice and these must harmonize with her facial expression. The nurse should be aware that after ten minutes of friendly persuasion with a confused patient, 'flashing' a look of despair or frustration at one of her colleagues may undo all the good she intended for the patient, as that particular fleeting message to someone else was the only thing understood by the patient! When success is achieved there is always a place for praise and other rewards, especially for those who achieve some measure of success in socially acceptable behaviour, i.e. eating, excreting and dressing habits. There is absolutely no place for pushing, pulling, ordering or shouting at such patients, or commanding that they should do as they are told. Kindness is the only effective approach, talking quietly and calmly, giving the impression, by your whole attitude, that you are the person who will help. Staying with the patients and allowing them to talk, however meaninglessly, often results in their developing a sense of relief and unburdening themselves—even if the following day once again escape is the only thing on their minds! For those patients who are unable to communicate verbally, touch has an important part to play in their care. For the nurse to sit and hold their hand or place an arm around their shoulder can increase their security and reduce their isolation.

Allocation of particular nurses to the total care of chosen individuals is more likely to result in the formation of some kind of helpful relationship. Nurses must make an effort to really get to know each patient in his own right. An attitude of respect and affection, attempting to identify what features of the remaining personality you like, will bring rewards in co-operation. The nurse should try to find out, by listening to the patient and talking to the relatives, something of his or her past achievements; very often the patient has made a greater contribution to the good of society than the nurse can ever expect to, or has had adventures, exploits and achievements in earlier life which are nothing short of impressive. Sometimes the patient will enjoy discussing his past pursuits. The patient should not become isolated because of his disability and the nurse should help to group similar patients together, hopefully so that some form of communication can take place.

The nurse should always try to assess the cause of restless behaviour in new and established patients. Discussion with colleagues may be fruitful, as may listening to the patient, even the patient whose utterings are usually of little meaning—he still has the right to speak and be heard. The nurse must remember that thirst, hunger, a full bladder and loaded rectum are all causes of restlessness. A urinary tract infection often leads to urethral and bladder irritation which makes the patient constantly seek a toilet he cannot find. He may tend to wander round the ward repeatedly appealing for help or asking for directions to his home.

The degree of distress suffered by the disorientated patient varies from day to day and from patient to patient. The new patient must, if possible, be housed away from exit doors and should not be permitted to worry heavily dependent, sick or dying patients. Because patients tend to wander about, a safe physical environment is essential. If the ward has obvious hazards nurses may be tempted to use a variety of restraints which eventually produce chairbound patients who cause no further trouble. Initially restraints in beds, i.e. cot sides, and in chairs to which tables are fixed, cause more frustration and restlessness. They are also more hazardous as the patients tend to climb over or under them. It may also be helpful to have various rooms such as the bathroom and lavatory identified by different coloured doors.

It is important that the nurse takes a pride in the appearance of her patients and the ward. Most patients are beyond being a credit to themselves, so the nursing team will be judged, fairly or not, by appearances.

Those patients who are dehydrated and refuse to drink are a challenge to the nurse. To offer drinks strictly on the hour is not a nurse's duty. Whenever the patient seems settled a drink should be offered and the amount charted. Trial and error with different drinks offered by nurses and relatives will often eventually prove successful. Fluid replacement by nasogastric tube or intravenously is notoriously unsuccessful with the confused patient.

Reality orientation
Reality orientation is now an accepted part of caring for the elderly and especially the elderly mentally infirm. In order to attempt to keep them orientated as to time, it is important to have the day, date and time clearly displayed in all parts of the ward, so that patients can read them where possible. The nurse must remember to check them daily, as it is doubly confusing if

dates etc. are not changed! Sometimes the weather and the season is visually displayed. In order to remind the elderly of friends and relatives, photographs and pictures should be encouraged, and this is often a good topic for conversation. Past hobbies and interests may be pursued if the patient is still able to grasp these. Simple games may be played, and well-known songs sung. Short sessions showing slides of local familiar landmarks may be helpful too. Making the ward as homelike as possible, even including a bar for drinks occasionally, may have a very beneficial effect on the patient!

Nursing the elderly mentally infirm requires skill, patience and understanding. It is often an unrewarding task as many of these patients are unable to express their gratitude and may not always be responsive. However it is a very essential part of nursing and many nurses enter into it with enthusiasm and humour.

References

Cox, J.R. (1983) Key vote for nurses in recognition of senile dementia. *Brit. J. Geriat. Nurs.* Vol. 3 (No. 2), p. 7.

Department of Health and Social Security (1981) *Growing Older.* London: HMSO.

Further reading

Altschul, A. & Simpson, R. (1984) *Psychiatric Nursing*, 6th edition. London: Baillière Tindall.

Burr, J. & Andrews, J. (1981) *Nursing the Psychiatric Patient*, 4th edition. London: Baillière Tindall.

Norman, A. (1982) *Mental Disease in Old Age.* London: Centre for Policy on Ageing.

Pitt, B. (1974) *Psychogeriatrics: An Introduction to the Psychiatry of Old Age.* Edinburgh: Churchill Livingstone.

11
Care of the Dying

Much of the work of the nurse when caring for the elderly is a positive, progressive approach to care, but it is inevitable because of the very nature of the work that a fairly high proportion of the patients will in fact die during the course of that care. Statistics show that in the assessment ward alone 30% of patients die within the first few weeks of admission, and at home a high proportion of patients die too. Although it may be stressful for the nursing staff, for some of the patients and for their relatives, it may also be a welcome relief from many years of disablement and chronic disease.

Much is currently written about caring for the dying and relief of pain, and with the increase in the hospice movement more attention is paid to the dying and their care. A 6-week course is currently run by the English National Board of Nursing Studies entitled 'Care of the Dying Patient and his Family' and this subject is included in the nurse's training programme. However, it is still regarded by many as a subject that should not be discussed and the care of those patients dying in hospital is often relegated to the side wards, where they may die in isolation and loneliness. Added stress is caused to the nursing staff as there is little time to grieve and many staff may have looked after the elderly for some time and developed firm relationships with them.

Care at home

Ideally most elderly people should die at home in surroundings familiar to them and with those they love around them. However, about 75% of people in the United Kingdom die in an institution away from home, and for the elderly the figure must be even higher than this as many of them are already living in institutions. No patient should be brought into hospital just to die, but many die there having failed to respond to treatment. Most people prefer to die in their own homes and the difficulty arises when there are not adequate carers to support them. Many live alone and their own relatives are themselves too old to cope with the care involved.

The following services are available:

1   The community nursing service is available for many but often not able to give the total care required.

2   The twilight and night nursing service is run by the community nursing service and looks after people requiring care at night on an intermittent basis. Some health authorities will provide a night sitter but it is often not a reliable service.

3   Home care teams consist of a specialist doctor and nurses who will advise and support the community nurses looking after those who are dying at home but do not offer practical nursing care. These nurses may be funded partly by voluntary subscription with help from the health authority, and in some cases by the National Society for Cancer Relief. One of the founders was Douglas Macmillan, so the nurses are known as Macmillan nurses.

4   The Marie Curie Foundation will sometimes pay for a night nursing service for those who are dying of cancer. It may also provide a sitter or pay for a night sitter from an agency.

5   Home help and laundry services provided by social services departments offer invaluable support to the carers at home.

6   Voluntary help is often available through Age Concern for sitting or helping with shopping, etc. Some group practices have now set up voluntary groups too who will help with these activities.

Hospice care

The development of hospices in various parts of the country has meant a small revolution in the care of those dying of a terminal illness. Dame Cicely Saunders founded St Christopher's Hospice in 1967 and through her inspiration much research has taken place into control of pain and the achievement of a peaceful and dignified death. Many hospices are financed wholly or partly by the local health authority and through voluntary subscription. It is an emotive subject and receives much public support. The hospice is usually small—30 to 40 beds—and provides a calm, relaxed atmosphere where those who are terminally ill can live their lives to the full until the end, when they can be confident in a peaceful death surrounded by family and friends. Most hospices provide intermittent care, so that patients can come in for assessment of their drug regimen and the relatives can be relieved for a short period. In many areas home support teams are attached to the hospice.

Hospital care

Many of the elderly die in the acute and continuing care wards of the geriatric unit as well as in the acute medical wards. Despite the fact that they may well be past their 'three score years and ten', they will need much physical and psychological support, as will their friends and relatives. The care should adequately reflect their needs and the nurse should spend time assessing her priorities. She needs to spend time also gaining the confidence of her patient as he may be reluctant to reveal his fears of pain, financial worries and fears of the unknown.

Physical needs

Much of the care given is similar to that required by any seriously ill patient. In order to care fully for the patient, individual wishes should be observed. Most discomforts can be relieved by a combination of good nursing and co-operation from the doctor.

Bathing
This should be carried out as normal. Some may prefer to be touched and moved as little as possible and these wishes must be observed; others may delight in a long soaking in a warm bath.

Pressure areas
To inflict the pain of pressure sores on a dying patient is an indignity best avoided. Routine care should be carried out, dry skin should be kept moist if possible with the aid of creams, and various devices may be used for relief of pressure, including the water bed, ripple bed, sheepskin, and various pressure-relieving mattresses and cushions (see Chapter 7).

Mouth care
This is important, especially as many drugs cause a dry mouth. Normal cleaning with toothbrush and toothpaste should

obviously be observed but frequent cleaning with glycerin and thymol or glycerin and borax helps to keep the mouth fresh. Some patients appreciate mouth swabs soaked with lemon and glycerin but these are inclined to be sickly. Dry lips respond well to bland creams and lipsalve. Refreshing, slightly acid drinks, sipping iced water or sucking ice cubes all help. Monilial infection (thrush) often occurs, especially in those patients on antibiotics. It is best treated with oral nystatin suspension rinsed around the mouth and then swallowed—1 ml 4-hourly. It can be prevented by sucking amphotericin lozenges.

Dyspnoea

This can be relieved by good positioning, nursing the patient either upright in bed with pillows placed in an 'armchair', or in a chair so that he can remain comfortably upright; the Buxton chair is very useful here. Most of these patients do not tolerate oxygen well and prefer a fan or an open window. A little sedation in the form of diazepam may be given and bronchial dilators may help in some cases. Where carcinoma of the bronchus is extensive an elixir of morphine or diamorphine will give good relief. Cough should be controlled where possible as it can be annoying to others as well as to the patient—a warm drink or linctus in hot water is often effective. Where there is difficulty expectorating mucus, an inhalation or the administration of bromhexine (Bisolvon), which loosens mucus, is helpful. Smoking should not be forbidden.

Nausea and vomiting

This is very common in patients suffering from terminal illness. It may be due to obstruction or bleeding from a growth, biochemical imbalance, or drugs and in some cases there may be a psychological element. Antiemetics in the form of the phenothiazines are most valuable early on and later cyclizine or metoclopramide may be added; these should be given a short while before a meal. Suitable and acceptable drinks should be given; again ice may be sucked as this keeps the mouth fresh and moist.

Anorexia

This is one of the most common symptoms of malignant disease and a little sherry before meals can be a good aperitif.

Prednisolone in small doses may also help, and the nurse can do much by presenting small appetizing looking meals which may tempt the patient to eat.

Dysphagia

This can be one of the most distressing symptoms of terminal disease. The nurse should offer food that she knows can be swallowed most easily, whether it is in the form of liquids or semi-solids, each patient having individual treatment. Most patients will require mild sedation to relieve distress, and mouth care to prevent any infection.

Insomnia

This is often encountered and the nurse should attend to the simple necessities of the patient before resorting to sedatives. She should ensure that the patient is comfortable, that the bowels and bladder are not full, that the patient is well positioned on the correct side, and that he is warm enough. Many patients suffer from poor peripheral circulation and require bedsocks or a hot-water bottle, provided it is not filled with boiling water and is adequately protected to avoid burns. An additional bedjacket, mittens, an extra soft blanket next to the body or a foam-backed synthetic fleece underblanket may all be helpful. A warm soothing drink with a little alcohol such as brandy and warm milk may be welcomed. A quiet chat with the nurse will be welcomed too. Finally, any pain must obviously be relieved and the ward kept quiet and peaceful. If all else fails a mild sedative or hypnotic may be used.

Bowels and bladder

These will need routine care. If the patient becomes incontinent of urine there are no contra-indications to catheterization for the terminally ill, and this may relieve restlessness and discomfort from an over-distended bladder or a perpetually wet bed. Emepronium may relieve those who suffer from frequency. Bowels should be observed and relieved where necessary with an enema or glycerol suppositories. A gentle laxative such as Senokot or Dorbanex may prove helpful—often the patient has his own favourite brand. This aspect of dying is often overlooked by the nursing staff and can cause much distress. An adequate diet containing bran and a good fluid intake can do much to relieve this distress.

Relief of pain

The relief of pain is a difficult aspect of the care of the dying, but nevertheless a very important one. Pain is not always well controlled, due partly to an inadequate understanding of its nature and partly to ill-founded fears of the 'addictive' nature of narcotic analgesics. Chronic pain, as experienced in terminal illness, is totally absorbing to the patient and results in isolation, depression, anxiety and fear. Addiction does not tend to occur where the pain is well controlled. Analgesics should be given regularly 4-hourly; the nurse should not wait for the pain to recur and the patient to demand a repeat dose. Mild pain can be relieved with aspirin, codeine, paracetamol or dextropropoxyphene, 2 tablets administered 4-hourly. Moderate pain can be controlled with 1–2 Diconal tablets 4-hourly or morphine or diamorphine elixir 5–10 mg 4-hourly with an added phenothiazine to act as an antiemetic and tranquillizer.

Severe pain may be controlled by morphine elixir 20–60 mg 4-hourly and if necessary diamorphine may be given by injection. Every patient is an individual and the dose of analgesic will vary. Some may require a considerably increased amount. The development of MST Continus—a slow-release morphine sulphate tablet which lasts for 12 hours—has made administration of analgesics easier for nurse and patient. It is produced in four different dosages and the tablets have to be swallowed whole. Bone pain is often difficult to control, but may be aided by the addition of an anti-inflammatory drug to other analgesics such as aspirin or ibuprofen.

Psychological needs

Security and companionship are two of the primary needs of the dying and so often the latter is denied to those who die in hospital. Loneliness of the dying patient can be severe. The patient is often nursed in a side ward away from other patients and therefore cut off from the activities of a busy ward, which in some cases can bring comfort. Nursing staff may tend to avoid these patients through fear and anxiety that they may be asked questions they cannot answer. The patients must have confidence in those caring for them and time must be given to them to relate their symptoms even if they are already known, and the nurse must be prepared to spend some time just listening to their fears and anxieties. So often, no advice or help is sought from the nurse, only a sympathetic ear. Passive listening can produce great relief of stress. Active listening too may be necessary and great skill is needed in asking questions and so encouraging the patient to talk. At least 25% of patients know that they are dying, and for the elderly it may be a relief from long suffering, loneliness and the discomfort of later life. The majority of elderly patients have a different approach to death from that of younger patients. The truth may have dawned on them without their being told, and they may not wish to discuss this. The art of listening is something to be learnt by all those who work in this field. On the whole patients are anxious only when they do not know their future but are at peace when they know that death is near.

Care of the dying involves team-work between the family, doctors, nurses, and the clergy because spiritual beliefs must be respected and their help should be sought from an early stage. Religious belief is obviously relevant when considering death and those with faith often die with less anxiety and apprehension. The clergy too are often helpful in relieving the anxieties of the family and the staff. The family should be encouraged to visit frequently, but short visits are often preferable to long visits as the latter can cause anxiety to the patient, the family's strains and stresses having been transmitted to them. The family should be prepared by the nursing staff for the deterioration in the patient, so that they do not become alarmed if the patient becomes disorientated or aggressive. The family will need much support from all the team during this stressful period; after the death of the patient this support will be given by the social worker, family doctor and health visitor. The nurse should find out at an early stage whether the relative wishes to be called at night should the patient deteriorate or die. When the patient has died, discretion should be exercised in informing the relatives. If they live alone, it may be done through the police, family doctor or a close friend. Some relatives like to view the patient after death, and this may be arranged either in the mortuary chapel or in the chapel of the funeral director.

When the patient is dying at home the relatives will need much support, looking after the patient 24 hours per day. When looking after a young family too the demands and strains may be great, and help may be necessary from voluntary and statutory sources.

In homes and hospitals where the elderly have lived for some time, they have formed close relationships with other residents and patients, and these friends may need much support from the nursing staff. Often when they are able, the friends like to help care for their companions.

Last offices

When the patient has died, the doctor should be notified immediately and will confirm that death has actually taken place. The nurse should then lay the patient flat, straighten all the limbs, clean the mouth and position the false teeth, bind the jaw, close the eyes with damp cotton wool and cover the patient with a sheet, having stripped the rest of the bed of bedding. All pillows, air rings, etc. should be removed, and any tubes should also be removed except in exceptional circumstances. The patient may then be left for up to one hour.

The final care of the patient should be administered by two nurses, one of whom should be senior and experienced in this work. The bed should be well screened off so that no one can possibly see the patient. The nurse will wash the patient, plugging the rectum, and the vagina in the female patient, and placing sleek or waterproof plaster over any open sores. The body is dressed in a suitable gown and clearly labelled, before being placed in a mortuary sheet and removed to the mortuary. All the patient's possessions should be listed and packed up, to be stored safely, preferably in the administrative offices. Valuables should be checked and locked away to await collection by the relatives.

The dignity of the patient should be preserved at all times. When the patient dies at home the relatives may be pleased to help with the last offices.

Bereavement

When caring for the dying patient, one must also remember the relatives and the aftercare of them once the patient has died. Time must be given to listening to their problems, worries and anxieties. All too often, once the funeral is over, the elderly relative is neglected and it is important that they are continued to be cared for, whether it is by the health visitor or by a voluntary visitor if there are no family around to help. If preparation for bereavement is good before the patient actually dies, the difficulties encountered after death may not be so severe. For the elderly the sense of loss and loneliness is often increased as they may have been together for very many years. This sense of loss may continue for many months and the aftercare should continue for as long as it is needed. In some areas bereavement counselling services have been set up and there is a branch of Cruse (a national organization for widows and widowers) in many towns.

Further reading

Copperman, H. (1983) *Dying at Home*. Chichester: John Wiley (An HM & M Nursing Publication).

Hinton, J. (1967) *Dying*. Harmondsworth: Penguin.

Nursing—The Add-on Journal of Clinical Nursing. Feb. 1982—Coping with Death.

Parkes, C.M. (1975) *Bereavement. Studies of Grief in Adult Life*. Harmondsworth: Penguin.

Purcell, W. (1978) *A Time to Die*. Mowbrays Popular Christian Paperbacks.

Robbins, J. (1983) *Caring for the Dying Patient and the Family*. London: Harper & Row.

Speck, P. (1978) *Loss and Grief in Medicine*. London: Baillière Tindall.

12
Further Care of the Elderly

At the present time in Great Britain some of the services provided for the elderly are theirs as a right, and these include access to health care and payment to almost all elderly of a pension. Locally some pensioners also have a right to free bus passes and other concessions. Since as early as 1536 there has been legislation to give help to the 'poor, impotent, lame, feeble, sick and diseased persons' under the old Poor Laws. Such help was often given grudgingly and the receipt of it implied a social stigma. The passing of the National Assistance Act 1948, which has been brought up to date by the Chronically Sick and Disabled Persons Act 1970, lays a duty on local authorities to provide such help as will be discussed in this chapter and seeks to dispel the idea that assistance is 'charity'. However, this idea does persist in the minds of many of the elderly who remember the old days of the workhouses.

Today the major duty of providing help for the disabled is undertaken by the State, but there is a big role for voluntary bodies, working with the statutory bodies. It is estimated that by 1991, there will be three million elderly in this country living alone and of these more than 5% will be both alone and unable to care for themselves adequately. Since the passing of the Chronically Sick and Disabled Persons Act in 1970, local authorities have been required to keep a register of disabled persons in their areas and by far the largest group of blind, deaf and otherwise handicapped persons are 65 years of age and over.

Statutory bodies

The two main statutory bodies responsible for the care of the elderly are the health authority and the social services department of the local authority. The health authority covers aspects of domiciliary care including home nurses and health visitors, so that preventive medicine is just as important as caring for the sick. The social services department is responsible for all aspects of social work both in the community and in hospital. The community nurses, health visitors and some social workers are also attached to the family practitioner service so that the services are closely bound together, the general practitioner often being the first point of contact with the elderly. The community nurse will carry out any necessary practical nursing procedures. The health visitor will visit those elderly persons referred to her by the general practitioner; ideally she would visit all old people on the practice list, but because of the size of her case load and the diversity of her work it is usually possible to keep only those known to be at risk under regular supervision. In some areas a health visitor may be attached to a geriatric unit and will visit the patient before his admission to hospital, during his stay there and after his discharge. Again, in some areas health visitors or registered nurses are employed to look after elderly patients only, the accent being on preventive medicine.

The care and welfare of the elderly is also one of the responsibilities of the social services departments of local authorities. Their aim is to keep people in their own homes for as long as possible, and to this end they are empowered to provide a number of services not only within people's own homes but within the community as well. Joint services with the health authority are common, e.g. day centres.

Housing

Housing of the elderly is obviously of great importance. Each local authority provides various types of accommodation, including independent flatlets, groups of flatlets in which there is a warden to keep an eye on the elderly and summon help when necessary, and residential accommodation. In the latter are housed old people who are able to get up and dress (although perhaps needing assistance), have a reasonable degree of mobility and can eat a meal without help. Those who are too frail to manage these minimum requirements are the responsibility of the National Health Service and may need to be cared for in continuing care units (see Chapter 4).

For some the ideal form of housing for the elderly is living with the family and yet having separate facilities. However, it is not in every family that this can be achieved, and many old people are fiercely independent and may refuse to live with the family even though there may be an obvious need for them to do so. Many old people still live in grossly inadequate and unsuitable accommodation, presenting a problem which may tax the ingenuity and resources of the social services.

Residential accommodation

Many old people who are not able to live alone do *not* require a hospital bed, but *do* require residential accommodation providing minimal care and attention. Most people decide of their own accord that they want to move into a home and at present there are over half a million old people living in such institutions in this country voluntarily. Under the National Assistance Act 1948, Section 47, certain powers are given to the District Medical Officer to arrange the removal of persons needing care and attention who suffer grave chronic disease or, being aged and infirm or physically handicapped, live in insanitary conditions and are unable to give themselves, and do not receive, proper care and attention. Application must be made to the magistrates and a limited period in care is applied which may be extended.

The National Health Service Act 1946, the National Assistance Act 1948 and Mental Health Act 1959 state that local authorities must provide residential accommodation for mentally and physically handicapped people and the elderly. Under Part III of the National Assistance Act, the needs for residential accommodation for the elderly are considered. This is provided by the local authority in homes of their own, or in homes managed by voluntary organizations, or in private homes registered for the purpose; the latter two sorts of home receive some financial aid from the local authority. Under the Residential Homes Act 1980, all private homes for the elderly or disabled must be registered with the local authority so that they can be inspected to see that they are properly equipped and maintained at a reasonable standard. All these homes should aim to provide a homely atmosphere and to meet the material needs of residents by providing nourishing food, adequate clothing and comfortable furnishings with recreational facilities including books, periodicals, newspapers, radio and television. The home should also provide a secure environment where the resident can feel he belongs and is cared for, so that he can face a crisis knowing he will have support and comfort from the staff. It should also maintain the resident's dignity, offering privacy and independence and acknowledging the resident's background and previous life-style as an important factor in his future. The residents should be encouraged to express their feelings on all aspects of their care. Staff should also provide such nursing care as would be given by relatives in their own home, the help of the community nurse being enlisted where necessary. The accommodation is not always ideal as suitable houses are not always available; but now, specially designed homes are being built which are well planned and have appropriate facilities. Finding and keeping suitable staff is often a problem.

All persons provided with residential accommodation must pay. If unable to pay the standard rate, they are assessed according to income, always being allowed to keep some pocket-money.

Some patients after a period of hospitalization may be unable to return to their own homes for a variety of reasons. The patient may now be too frail physically or unstable mentally to be able to live alone. The relations with whom he may have been living, having enjoyed a period of freedom while their relative was in hospital, are now reluctant to resume their responsibilities. Whatever the reason, the thought of going into a home is regarded with great misgivings by the majority of patients. Loss of independence, personal possessions and a home of their own and, even more, the loss of privacy on entering into a communal life, are thoughts not welcome to many elderly persons. Much hard work has to be done by the whole team, specially the nursing staff, social worker and chaplain, who have most opportunity to talk quietly to the patient. The decision should be made slowly; it is not something to be rushed into, and patients should be made to feel that they themselves, and not the hospital authorities or their relatives, have made the decision. Co-operation and support will be sought from the relatives who should also be closely involved in the selection of the home. Choice of a suitable home is all important to the future happiness of the elderly person. An assessment of the patient's income will be made and the value of the patient's house, if there is one, will be properly assessed, as places in local authority homes are few and vacancies in private homes easier to come by. Some people like communal life with plenty of people around; some prefer more seclusion with opportunity to pursue their own hobbies and interests.

There are three categories of old people's homes: local authority, voluntary and private.

Local authority homes   Residential accommodation provided by the local authority varies from old houses, including old workhouses converted into homes, to modern purpose-built houses with lifts and other modern devices. The atmosphere, so important to maintain the morale of the residents, will depend almost entirely upon the head of home and her staff. The homes are graded as follows:

1   For the physically frail—grade A for those needing little help or care, grade B for those needing considerably more care and attention.
2   For the mentally frail; those who are mentally precarious and therefore require much more help on the whole.

Grading is necessary so that adequate staff can be provided to help the residents. It is important that when application is made for a place in these homes, a true picture of the resident's ability is given, so that he is correctly placed and can receive sufficient help. When an application has been made, a social worker from the community will visit the resident to assess his ability and suitability to enter a home and to ask the resident for his consent for his name to be put forward. They may also discuss the selling of the resident's own property and the disposal of his effects. Many homes do make provision for residents to take their own ornaments, crockery and a table or chair if they particularly desire this. Meanwhile it is often possible for the social worker or relatives to take the resident to visit a home, so that he can see in advance where he is going. Often the resident is adamant that he does not wish to go, but returns from such a visit with a completely different view of communal life. Before the resident finally goes to a home, he is generally visited by the head of home so that he sees at least one familiar face when he arrives. The home is notified of the approximate time of arrival so that a good welcome can be assured, and it is best if either a relative or social worker can accompany the resident. It is usually best for a resident to go into a home directly from the geriatric unit, so that he has had time for readjustment and has reached his maximum mobility and fitness. If the time spent waiting for a vacancy is too long, the resident can easily deteriorate and no longer qualify for the home proposed.

Voluntary homes These include convents, Salvation Army homes, Women's Royal Voluntary Service homes, Abbeyfield homes and some homes for those with special needs. Much research is now being done by such associations into the types of homes required by the elderly, and more emphasis is being put on flatlets rather than communal homes. Again, careful selection is needed by the social worker for these types of homes. For instance, one would hesitate before suggesting that an atheist or agnostic should go to live in a convent or Salvation Army home, which is obviously appropriate for those who share the convictions of the staff.

Private residential homes These vary from guest-houses to residential care homes where a fairly adequate amount of care is given. Most are run by the owners and are fairly abundant in areas where there is a high proportion of elderly people in the community. These may be better for those who prefer more privacy and less of a communal life. They are generally smaller and often do not enjoy all the amenities of the local authority homes. The Department of Health and Social Security may now contribute a substantial amount to the cost of the elderly living in private homes.

Most homes arrange some social activities, often in conjunction with a local school or youth club. The young people visit and organize communal games. Outings may be possible, and visits to local shops and theatres and even holidays can be arranged. The local clergy should call and hold services or arrange for the residents to attend local church services. Relatives are normally encouraged to visit as often as possible and even take the residents out for the day or weekend. Many homes now have a residents' committee which is responsible for organizing the social activities of the home.

All private and voluntary homes are inspected by the local services department in accordance with the 1980 Residential Homes Act. This applies to homes for disabled persons, old people's homes and residential homes for the mentally disordered. The inspection should include the building, provision of meals and recreation for the residents.

Nursing homes These homes are privately owned and are

registered with the local health authority under the Nursing Homes Act 1975. They include any home providing nursing for any person suffering from any sickness, injury or infirmity and are inspected by the health authority at least twice yearly. They are required to provide adequate space and equipment, and for a Registered General Nurse to be on the premises 24 hours per day. In 1984 amendments have been made to allow for dual registration of homes, so that nursing needs of residents in residential homes can be met as they become more frail and ill.

Financial assistance

It is important that the nurse is aware of the many grants and benefits available to the elderly and disadvantaged.

1 National Insurance benefits
These can be claimed by the elderly (or sometimes their spouse) if they have paid enough National Insurance contributions. They are not subject to a means test and are reviewed annually, being adjusted to the rate of inflation. The main benefits under this heading which affect the elderly are:
a   retirement pension
b   invalidity benefit
c   widow's allowance
d   widow's pension
e   death grant.

2 Means-tested benefits
No National Insurance contributions are required but the benefits are means tested. This entails giving details of both capital and income, and if the capital exceeds the statutory limit (£3000 as at September 1984) no benefit will be payable. Total income is deducted from total requirements as calculated in accordance with the limits laid down by Parliament which are reviewed annually. If the requirements exceed resources, then a supplementary pension is payable.

Under this heading the main benefits are:
a   supplementary benefit—beneficiaries automatically receive free prescriptions, free glasses, free dental help and help with hospital fares
b   rent rebates and allowances
c   rate rebates.

3 *Non-contributory benefits*

These benefits do not depend on National Insurance contributions or on the elderly's income, but do depend on their state of health and may be affected by any injuries previously suffered at work. They include:

a   attendance allowance, i) for those needing care 24 hours per day, and ii) for those needing care only during the day

b   invalid care allowance—given to a person of working age who is required to look after an elderly person already in receipt of an attendance allowance

c   mobility allowance—given before the age of 65 years but payable until the age of 75 years

d   industrial disability benefit—if injured at work or for one of the prescribed industrial diseases

e   industrial death benefit—if death results from an accident at work, dependants may claim

f   over 80 pension—for people over 80 who are not entitled to a pension or only a very small pension.

4 *Other help and services*

Where age has led to handicap or other disadvantage other benefits are available either in cash or kind. These include:

a   aids, equipment and adaptations
b   help with holidays
c   home help
d   meals-on-wheels
e   special housing
f   laundry services
g   installation and rental of television
h   installation and rental of telephone
i   advice from social worker
j   residential accommodation
k   day hospitals
l   day centres.

5 *General advice*

When help is required of either a financial or material nature, it is wise to ask what help is available and consult the social services department. The benefits system is complex, as are some of the conditions for the granting of these benefits. If a benefit requested is refused this will be notified in writing but there is a right to appeal, usually within 30 days. The letter of appeal should be clear, stating the condition of the patient, what help is needed, and for how long this has been so.

Legal arrangements

It is necessary for the nurse to be aware of legal assistance available to protect the property and affairs of those elderly people who are unable to administer them for themselves.

Power of attorney

This is a legal arrangement whereby one person empowers another to manage his affairs. It may be in general form, granting power to manage all affairs all the time, or specific power may be granted over some matters under specified circumstances. This power cannot be granted by a person suffering mental disability (see below under Court of Protection). In order to be valid it must be stamped by the Inland Revenue. If a person who has given the power subsequently suffers mental disability, the power becomes void. The document should be witnessed by an independent person, preferably a doctor or solicitor.

Court of Protection

The Court of Protection is concerned with the protection of the property of persons who, because of mental disorder, are incapable of managing their own affairs. This protection covers all patients who have property or an income, whether they are in hospital, in a home or living in their own home. When a person suffers a mental disability, he cannot give a power of attorney or any other authority to someone else to manage his affairs, and until authority has been obtained from the Court of Protection there is no-one able to act on behalf of the patient. Application to the court should always be made through a solicitor.

Legal aid

If a patient is on a low income, help may be available whenever it is necessary to see a solicitor for legal advice and assistance, or whenever legal aid is needed for court cases. The benefit is means tested and provides for legal advice free or at a low cost up to a cash limit. Legal aid for court cases may be subject to the patient making a financial contribution, but can cover the work done by a solicitor up to and including the court proceedings and representation by a solicitor or barrister if necessary. It is available for both civil and criminal cases. Many solicitors also provide advice for up to half an hour for a comparatively small amount. This is not means tested.

From this review of some of the services that are available to old people from the family practitioner service, the National Health Service and the local authority social services department, as well as from the private sector, it will be seen that to ensure the best that can be provided for the old and disabled a high degree of liaison and good will between those who help them is a first priority.

Further reading

Brearley, C.P. (1975) *Residential Work and the Elderly*. London: Routledge and Kegan Paul.

Brearley, C.P. (1977) *Social Work, Ageing and Society*. London: Routledge and Kegan Paul.

DHSS (1983) *Which Benefit?* (leaflet FB2) London: HMSO.

Tinker, A. (1981) *The Elderly in Modern Society*. New York: Longman.

Appendix:
Equipment in the Geriatric Unit

It would clearly be impractical to attempt to describe all the
varieties of equipment which might be found in the geriatric
unit, as this will vary considerably from hospital to hospital.
However, the nurse in the unit will need to be familiar with the
general types of equipment and aids which are available, and
should know something about the functioning of at least the
most common types.

Beds

King's Fund bed　This is an adjustable height bed, operated
by a pump. The head and foot may operate separately. The
head is removable and the foot lets down to provide a rack for
stripping the bedclothes. The base is solid and a foam mattress
is used.

Nesbitt–Evans high–low bed　The height of this bed is also
adjustable, and the head and foot may be elevated separately by
means of a lever mechanism.

Water flotation bed　This comprises a flexible membrane for
the mattress, supported by a fibreglass tank on a mobile steel
structure.

Net suspension bed　This consists of a nylon mesh net
attached to two turning poles which can be attached to a King's
Fund bed.

Bedcradles

Harborough bedcradle　The cradle consists of a strong,
chromium-plated steel tube. One end fits under the mattress
and the other takes the weight of the bedclothes.

Hoists

Ambulift   This lift has a variety of uses, the main purpose being to lift the patient in and out of the bath. It is very stable, as the seat is fixed and there are arm rests, and it gives the patient firm security. It can be taken to the bedside and used to help the patient out of bed. The seat can be detached and placed on separate wheels. A bedpan attachment allows it to be used as a commode. If it is necessary to move an exceptionally heavy patient in and out of bed, there are sling attachments, which are very helpful.

Chairs

Many types of chairs are available, and it is wise to have as large a selection as possible on the ward to accommodate a variety of patients.

Fountain chair   This is a straightforward chair with a back 112 cm (44 in) high and a seat 46 cm (18 in) high. It is vinyl-covered and the arms come well forward.

Tyne chair   This is similar to the Fountain, but has in addition a swivel tray which can be fixed on at a convenient place. The chair may be made mobile by gripping the bars together behind the backrest. This raises the rear chair legs and the whole chair may be pushed forwards.

Easy-to-rise chair   This chair is designed for the many old people who find it difficult to rise from an ordinary low chair. The chair legs are splayed out and tipped with rubber to give maximum stability. The angle of the back may be altered and the seat height may be adjusted from 46 cm (18 in) to 60 cm (24 in). The arms project 23 cm (9 in) beyond the front of the seat to provide extra leverage when rising. The covering is washable.

Self-lift chair   This chair has a spring attachment under the seat so that the patient is gently eased up from it. It is useful for patients who have a physical disability which makes it difficult for them to rise initially.

Buxton chair   This is another mobile chair, ideal for the more seriously ill patient who needs greater support. The chair may be tipped backwards through a wide angle, enabling the patient to sleep comfortably if necessary.

Parker-Knoll chair   This is upright and makes it easy for the elderly person to rise.

Adjustable lavatory seats and frames

Seat-aid   This is a strong but light steel tube frame which fits round any free-standing lavatory. It has non-slip feet and plastic grips which assist the patient to sit and rise safely.

Plastic seat-aid   This is a plastic seat which fits directly into the pan and raises the seat by 10 to 15 cm (4 to 6 in).

Adjustable height toilet seat   This is a chromium-plated tube frame with moulded plastic arm rests, which enables the seat to be adjusted to the correct height.

Bath aids

Economic bath safety rail   This can be fitted to any bath with conventional taps. Rubber handgrips prevent slipping. It can be moved away above the taps when not in use.

Projecting bath bench and seat   This is designed for those who experience difficulty getting in and out of the bath, owing to weakness or stiffness.

Non-slip bathmat   If placed in the bottom of the bath this reduces the dangers of the patient slipping on the enamel. It is kept in position by rubber suction cups.

Dressing-aids

Lazy tongs   These assist dressing generally, and are useful for reaching.

Long-handled shoehorn   This is again useful for patients who have difficulty reaching their feet.

Elastic laces   These are useful for patients who have to dress using only one hand, or who cannot easily reach their feet.

Stocking gutter   If the patient cannot reach her feet this will be of great assistance in pulling on stockings.

Feeding-aids

Cutlery handles   Rubazote sponge tubing is available in six gauges for those who have difficulty in gripping narrow handles.

Manoy cutlery   This is useful for patients who find it difficult to reach their mouths, e.g. in parkinsonism or rheumatoid arthritis.

Nelson knife   This knife combines the action of knife and fork; food is cut by a rocking motion on the curve of the blade. It is particularly useful for the hemiplegic patient.

Plate bunker   A plastic or Perspex buffer fitted with riveted spring clips which will fit a plate of any reasonable size.

Non-slip mats   These mats, which may be made of plastic foam, pimple rubber or plastic webbing, are essential for the disabled.

Manoy crockery   Melaware make this range of crockery specifically for the disabled.

Walking-aids

Walking-frame   A frame made of light alloy tubing provides stable but lightweight support between steps for the patient who is mobile but unsteady.

Rollator   This frame does not need to be lifted right off the ground between steps, but nor does it run away with the user. It is often useful for those with parkinsonism.

Tripod or quadriped   Walking-sticks with tripod or quad-riped bases, made of lightweight tubular steel with rubber feet, give more support than ordinary walking-sticks and are useful for the hemiplegic.

Index